SSSP

Springer
Series in
Social
Psychology

SSSP

The Social Psychology of Intergroup Conflict

Theory, Research and Applications

Edited by
Wolfgang Stroebe   Arie W. Kruglanski
Daniel Bar-Tal   Miles Hewstone

Springer-Verlag Berlin Heidelberg New York
London Paris Tokyo

Wolfgang Stroebe
Psychologisches Institut, Universität Tübingen
7400 Tübingen, Federal Republic of Germany

Arie W. Kruglanski
Department of Psychology, University of Maryland
College Park, MD 20742, USA

Daniel Bar-Tal
School of Education, Tel-Aviv University
Tel-Aviv 69978, Israel

Miles Hewstone
Department of Psychology, University of Bristol
Bristol BS8 1HH, England

ISBN 3-540-17695-0 Springer-Verlag Berlin Heidelberg New York
ISBN 0-387-17695-0 Springer-Verlag New York Berlin Heidelberg

Library of Congress Cataloging-in-Publication Data
The Social psychology of intergroup conflict. (Springer series in social psychology) Includes indexes.
1. Intergroup relations. 2. Conflict management. I. Stroebe, Wolfgang. II. Series.
HM291.S58865 1988 302.3'4 87-23320
ISBN 0-387-17695-0 (U.S.)

Typesetting, printing and binding: G. Appl, Wemding
2126/3145-543210

Preface

The idea for this book was the result of a planned social intervention aimed at encouraging social relations between two groups, which, though not in conflict, previously had had very little contact. To correct an anomaly which had existed far too long, namely, the total lack of interaction between social psychologists from Europe and Israel, a meeting had been organized under the auspices of the European Association of Experimental Social Psychology and the Israeli Association of Social Psychology that took place in a kibbutz near Tel Aviv late in 1983. The theme of the meeting was formulated very broadly as "Group processes and intergroup conflict" to allow a selection of participants on the basis of quality rather than area of research.

To our surprise, this caution turned out to be unnecessary. The majority of the papers centered around the topic of conflict. However, while the European work on conflict relied heavily on experimental laboratory research, most of the Israeli research consisted of field studies, which frequently focused on the Israeli-Palestinian conflict.

If one considers the social context of European and Israeli social psychology, one begins to understand the reasons for both the similarities in topic as well as the differences in approach. European interest in the area of conflict had been stimulated by the late Henri Tajfel's work on the "minimal group paradigm" and his "social identity theory." There are many reasons why Tajfel's work caught the imagination of European social psychologists. It linked the study of intergroup relations to some of the cognitive work on categorization which had been popular in Europe during the early 1970s. It claimed to confront the individualistic social psychology predominant in the United States with a *social* social psychology. But most importantly, it offered the first theoretical development to support the claim that there were social psychologists in Europe who held a distinctly European perspective.

The reasons why Israeli social psychologists have been interested in conflict are more practical and less academic. Whether because of the smallness of the country and its political and economic situation, the pioneer spirit, or the aversion of Israeli scientists to ivory towers, Israeli social psychologists seemed to be constantly called upon to investigate and solve social problems by governmental agencies. Since Israel is a country that is not only in conflict with its Arab neighbors, but as a multiethnic society is also subject to internal conflicts and tensions, most of our Israeli colleagues at the conference seemed to have been intricately involved with different aspects of the manifold conflicts that trouble this society.

This difference in orientation, though sometimes endangering the political aim of this meeting, made for a fascinating conference. On the one hand, we had the European social psychologists who in their laboratories tested predictions (carefully derived from social identity theory) with groups whose only cause of quarrel had been an alleged difference in their preference for paintings of Klee and Kandinsky. On the other hand, we had the Israeli social psychologists, who negotiated with terrorists or tried to reduce conflicts between Arab and Jewish students at Israeli universities and schools. While this difference in perspective initially had all the makings of a new intergroup conflict (between the "atheoretical" and the "irrelevant" group), we were soon struck by the exciting complementarity that existed between European and Israeli approaches to conflict.

At this stage the idea for this volume was born. The editors envisaged a book that was to integrate these two perspectives. Since we wanted chapters that were *both* theoretical *and* socially relevant, none of the original conference presentations were included in this book. Instead, we asked some of the participants at that conference (as well as some other colleagues) to write chapters that offered theoretical analyses of important issues in the area of intergroup conflict. We hope that the collection of chapters in this book will convey some of the excitement that motivated us to undertake this task.

Wolfgang Stroebe
Arie W. Kruglanski
Daniel Bar-Tal
Miles Hewstone

Table of Contents

List of Contributors

Dr. Yehuda Amir
Department of Psychology, Bar-Ilan University, 52 100 Ramat Gan, Israel

Dr. Daniel Bar-Tal
School of Education, Tel-Aviv University, Tel-Aviv 69978, Israel

Dr. Rachel Ben-Ari
Department of Psychology, Bar-Ilan University, 52 100 Ramat Gan, Israel

Dr. Rupert Brown
Institute of Social and Applied Psychology, University of Kent, Canterbury, Kent CT2 7NS, England

Dr. Susan Condor
Department of Psychology, University of Lancaster, Fylde College, Bailrigg, Lancaster LA1 4YF, England

Dr. Nehemia Friedland
Department of Psychology, Tel-Aviv University, Ramat Aviv 69978, Tel-Aviv P.O.B. 39040, Israel

Dr. Miles Hewstone
Department of Psychology, University of Bristol, Bristol BS8 1HH, England

Dr. John E. Hofman
Department of Psychology, University of Haifa, Mount Carmel, Haifa 31999, Israel

Dr. Klaus Jonas
Psychologisches Institut, Universität Tübingen, 7400 Tübingen, Federal Republic of Germany

Dr. Yechiel Klar
School of Education, Tel-Aviv University, Tel-Aviv 69978, Israel

Dr. Arie W. Kruglanski
Department of Psychology, University of Maryland, College Park, MD 20742, USA

Dipl.-Psych. Andrea Lenkert
Psychologisches Institut, Universität Tübingen, 7400 Tübingen, Federal Republic of Germany

Dr. Waldemar Lilli
Fakultät für Sozialwissenschaften, Sozialpsychologie, Universität Mannheim, 6800 Mannheim 1, Federal Republic of Germany

Dr. Ariel Merari
Department of Psychology, Tel-Aviv University, Ramat Aviv 69978, Tel-Aviv, P.O.B. 39040, Israel

Dr. Ian E. Morley
Department of Psychology, University of Warwick, Coventry CV4 7AL, England

Dr. J. Rehm
Fakultät für Sozialwissenschaften, Sozialpsychologie, Universität Mannheim, 6800 Mannheim 1, Federal Republic of Germany

Dr. Geoffrey M. Stephenson
Institute of Social and Applied Psychology, University of Kent, Canterbury, Kent CT2 7NS, England

Dr. Wolfgang Stroebe
Psychologisches Institut, Universität Tübingen, 7400 Tübingen, Federal Republic of Germany

Dr. Janette Webb
Management Centre, University of Aston, Birmingham G4 7DU, England (present address: Department of Business Studies, University of Edinburgh, William Robertson Building, 50 George Square, Edinburgh EH8 9JY, Scotland)

Part I

Introduction

Chapter 1

Psychological Processes in Intergroup Conflict

Susan Condor and Rupert Brown

The existence of conflictual relations between social groups is a pervasive feature of human society. Whereas some forms of intergroup rivalry are socially condoned and even encouraged on the basis that they promote ingroup loyalty (team sports) and protect the democratic process (party politics), other manifestations of social conflict are regarded as highly pernicious. Indeed, it is notable that social psychologists have shown particular interest in intergroup conflict in those historical periods when this has been defined as a social problem (e. g., the persecution of the Jews, the Second World War, the intranational conflicts of the 1960s and 70s).

Our aim in this chapter is to examine some of the ways in which psychologists have viewed intergroup conflict. First we will outline some of the major theoretical perspectives in this field, although it is clearly beyond the scope of a single chapter to do justice to the decades of psychological theory and research relating to this issue; the interested reader is referred to the many excellent existing reviews (e. g. Brewer & Kramer, 1985; Tajfel, 1982a; Turner, 1984). We will then turn to consider the application of general psychological theories to particular instances of intergroup conflict.

Theoretical Perspectives

Intergroup Conflict as a Product of Universal Psychological Characteristics

The prevalence of social conflict has led many social theorists to seek the root of such hostility in some form of aggressive "drive" or "need" common to the human species (e. g., Lorenz, 1967; Simmel, 1955). This perspective is shared by psychologists, who, like McDougall (1919) have attributed collective combat to the operation of an "instinct of pugnacity." In particular, Freud's (e. g., 1921)

elaborate theory in which intergroup conflict was seen to derive from unconscious forces associated with the resolution of the Oedipus conflict has exerted
a profound influence on subsequent psychological theorizing (see, e.g., Durbin & Bowlby, 1938; Fromm, 1977; Roheim, 1950; Storr, 1968, for adaptations
of the original Freudian position).

Theories which account for intergroup conflict in terms of universal aggressive drives face problems in accounting for the *absence* of antagonism. It is not,
therefore, surprising that subsequent work in the Freudian tradition sought to
supplement the postulate of universal aggressive tendencies with an analysis of
the *particular* contexts in which hostility is actually engendered and displayed
towards an outgroup. The classic work of this genre, the frustration-aggression
hypothesis (F-A; Dollard, Miller, Doob, Mowrer, & Sears, 1939) attempted to
synthesize Freudian premises with constructs drawn from learning theory in order to explain the particular circumstances in which a universal aggressive
drive becomes operative (specifically in response to "frustrating" stimuli). This
perspective was later extended, notably by Berkowitz (1962, 1969) who suggested that symbols possessing learned associations with violence may act as relea-
sers for acts of aggression in certain circumstances. Collective conflict was seen
to result from the simultaneous exposure of a number of individuals to the
same frustrating stimuli. Dollard and his associates outlined the various forms
of frustration inherent in major political systems, and later elaborations of this
perspective have suggested that revolutions may occur when social structural
arrangements prevent a large number of individuals from achieving need-ful-
fillment (Davies, 1973).

Explanations of intergroup conflict in terms of aggressive drives generally
represent hostility as the product of "unreasoning and unreasonable human nature" (Lorenz, 1967, p. 228). Hence, Osgood (1962) refers to the "Neanderthal"
mentality prevalent in intergroup relations, and other writers draw an analogy
between the behavior of nations preparing for war and individual "maladaptive" behavior, such as anorexia and nocturnal enuresis (e.g., Davis, 1963).
Some have even speculated on the physiological bases for collective "irrationality," suggesting, for example, that during large-scale social conflict the cor-
tex loses control of the limbic system (Koestler, 1969).

In contrast, recent research has followed the work of early stereotyping theorists (Allport, 1954; Tajfel, 1969), suggesting that hostile intergroup attitudes
may be analyzed in terms of *normal* cognitive functioning involved in impression formation. This approach is exemplified by the "new" social cognition
perspective which aims to relate the ideological aspects of intergroup conflict
to recent advances in the understanding of "basic cognitive processes" (Hamilton, 1981).

While most social cognition research is confined to the analysis of individual information processing, Snyder and his colleagues (e.g., Snyder, 1981) have
considered the way in which stereotypes may be used and maintained in *inter*-
personal interaction. In this they share the orientation of another major approach to social conflict: that which considers the rational interpersonal processes operating in gaming situations as an analogy of intergroup conflict (e.g.,

Deutsch, 1973; Kelley, 1968; Rapoport, 1965). Of particular concern have been "mixed motive" games such as the Prisoner's Dilemma, studies of which have typically found that players become locked into competitive strategies although this is to their ultimate disadvantage (see, e.g., Eiser, 1980). The parallels between this laboratory context and the arms race have not been overlooked (Deutsch, 1973).

Detailed critiques of the Freudian, F-A, social cognition, and gaming perspectives as theories or analogues of intergroup conflict have been provided elsewhere (see, e.g., Ashmore & Del Boca 1976; Billig, 1976; Etzioni, 1969; Katz, 1961; Sherif, 1966; Tajfel, 1978a, 1979, 1982a). We will simply note some of the general problems associated with analyses of intergroup conflict in terms of universal psychological mechanisms.

On the theoretical level, a major conceptual problem concerns the schism which has developed between analyses focusing on the motivational and those concentrating on the cognitive aspects of intergroup hostility. It has already been noted how motivation theorists largely overlook cognitive processes. Conversely, despite the "new look" in perception research in Tajfel's early work which emphasized the need to regard motivation and perception as interrelated (see Tajfel, 1981a), social cognition researchers typically regard human information processing independently of motivational factors. Although there appears to be a trend towards the recognition of the potential importance of motivational factors in stereotyping, social cognition researchers still consider these to be factors which can be simply added on to a purely cognitive analysis of the phenomenon (see Pettigrew, 1981).

Second, approaches which seek to ground intergroup conflict in cognitive or motivational states tend to be highly individualistic, often overlooking the role of collective norms or social ideology in intergroup conflict. In this vein, Billig (1976) criticizes the Freudian perspectives which attempt to reduce intergroup conflict to the intra- and interindividual dynamics (see, in particular, Roheim's [1950] explicitly reductionist "ontogenetic" theory of culture), and Tajfel (1972, p. 105) questions the adequacy of the F-A hypothesis: "Shared social conduct is not shared because we are all frustrated; it is shared by those who have all accepted . . . the same theory of social causation."

Contemporary social cognition research specifically employs the isolated individual as its unit of analysis, even redefining the notion of "stereotype" as involving individual rather than collective representations of social groups (e.g., McCauley & Stitt, 1978). It is suggested that stereotypes have been defined consensually "not for any compelling theoretical reason, but because [the] methodology dictated the use of agreement among perceivers to [identify] stereotypes" (Ashmore & Del Boca, 1979, pp. 222–223). In contrast, we would suggest that there has been a very compelling theoretical reason behind efforts to study consensual beliefs about race, sex, and ethnic categories. Interest in these issues has been largely motivated by a desire to understand (and possibly eradicate) a prevalent social problem. Needless to say, hostile images of an outgroup only take on social importance because they are widespread (Gardner, 1973). Rather than it being the case that the "consensus" approach to stereotyping arose as an accidental by-product of the methodology employed, it seems more plausible to suggest that methodology such as that employed by Katz and Braly (1933) was actually devised in the first place to fit in with a preexisting notion of stereotypes as widely held.

Social cognition research tends to reduce not only the stereotyper but also the stereotyped to the level of the individual, typically focusing on the attribution of stereotypic characteristics to individual category members (e.g., Locksley, Hepburn, Borgida,&Brekke, 1980; Taylor, 1981), and often specifically relating this to work on person perception (e.g., Ashmore&Tumia, 1980; Hamilton, 1981). Approaches which distil the issue of stereotyping down to the problem of one individual's impression of another must overlook their role in inter*group* settings. It is well known that we often have no direct contact with members of groups about whom we hold negative stereotypes: none of Katz and Braly's subjects had ever met a Turk, and doubtless prior to March 1982 few British citizens had firsthand experience of Argentinians. It is, however, in such situations of minimal inter*personal* contact that stereotypes may exert most influence over intergroup conflict.

The explanation of intergroup conflict in terms of supposedly universal psychological processes may also be criticized on pragmatic grounds. The obvious question to arise from this work is why, if intergroup conflict is a natural and necessary aspect of human psychological functioning, individuals have to be coerced to fight in wars (see Klineberg, 1950; Sherif, 1966). Perhaps the most often criticized aspect of "psychological universal" explanations is their inherent pessimism: if conflict is rooted in "basic" and universal aspects of human psychology, what chance is there for conflict resolution? (see Billig, 1985, for a recent example; but see, e.g., Durbin&Bowlby, 1938; Storr, 1968, for denials of this charge). It is for these reasons that many psychologists have sought stable individual differences in the propensity to engage in hostile intergroup activity.

"Individual Differences" Approaches to Intergroup Conflict

Psychologists have, naturally, suggested that the "universal" motivational and cognitive processes associated with intergroup conflict may be subject to some degree of individual variation. People may, for example, differ in the strength of their response to frustrating stimuli (Himmelweit, 1950) or in their tendency to use particular systems of categorization (Bem, 1981). Most influential and systematic of the "individual differences" perspectives is clearly the attempt to analyze individual differences in Freudian processes which was initiated by Adorno and his colleagues (Adorno, Frenkel-Brunswick, Levinson,&Sanford, 1950), whose vast research program was directed towards the identification of particular individuals receptive to antisemitic ideology (the "potentially fascistic individual"). A great deal of work in the 1950s and 1960s was concerned with documenting the motivational and cognitive characteristics of the so-called authoritarian personality (categorical and stereotypic thought, conventionality, concern for power, obedience to authority, aggression, and punitiveness), and studying its origins in childrearing practices (see, e.g., Kirsch&Dillehay, 1967). Later theorists extended the perspective in order to demonstrate that individuals receptive to left-wing beliefs may be characterized by psychological dogmatism (Eysenck&Wilson, 1978; Rokeach, 1960; Shils, 1957).

With the rise of protest movements in the 1960s and 1970s, some researchers interested in individual differences shifted their emphasis from the analysis of the prejudice of majority group members towards attempts to account for subordinate group activity in terms of the personality characteristics of the participants, for example, analyzing the women's movement and the black civil rights protests in terms of the distinctive personality characteristics of their members (e.g., Cherniss, 1972; Crawford&Nadich, 1970; Forward&Williams, 1970; Kravetz, 1976).

Leaving aside methodoligical criticisms of particular approaches (see, e.g., Brown, 1965; Cherry&Byrne, 1977; Christie&Jahoda, 1954), an obvious argument against such an "individual differences" perspective is that intergroup conflict involves, by definition, not just particular individuals, but whole communities, "If intergroup behavior were first and foremost a matter of understanding the behavior of exceptionally disturbed individuals, it would not be the issue of vital consequence that it is today" (Sherif, 1966, p. 13). As Milner (1981) notes, the very notion of the authoritarian as an *abnormal* or disturbed individual precludes attempts to use this phenomenon to explain racial prejudice in the USA or apartheid in South Africa. Personality theorists have tackled the problem of *widespread* social conflict in two main ways. First, they have developed the original assumption outlined in *The Authoritarian Personality* (Adorno et al. 1950) that certain personality structures may be fostered in particular social climates (e.g., economic conditions accompanied by pervasive social ideologies concerning childrearing practices), leading to the analysis of "national character" – the distinctive personality characteristics typifying a whole nation and accounting for its common action (e.g., Dicks, 1950). The obvious problem with such approaches is their inability to account for intragenerational or intranational fluctuations in the pervasiveness of prejudice or conflict (Pettigrew, 1958), and, further, why those nations characterized by authoritarian personality structures have not, in fact, been those involved in the most social conflict (see Sherif, 1966). Alternatively, theorists have attempted to account for widespread social conflict with recourse to the distinctive psychological characteristics of particular individuals holding positions of social influence and power (e.g., Herman&Herman, 1982). However, this implies a view of leadership which is reminiscent of the by now generally discredited trait theory (see Stogdill, 1974), and is not readily compatible with current perspectives which emphasize the contingent or reciprocal nature of the leadership process (e.g., Fiedler, 1967; Hollander, 1978).

In order to understand the psychological processes associated with intergroup conflict, it is clearly necessary to consider the interrelationship between cognition and motivation (as the authoritarian personality authors do), whilst also recognizing that the widespread nature of human conflict suggests that these must represent normal rather than pathological processes (as the social cognition workers do). The fact that the cognitive and motivational processes associated with intergroup conflict must be regarded as widespread need not imply that they are always operative, and it is important to consider *when* it is that these psychological processes actually come into operation (as the F-A theorists do). We will now consider two perspectives which have laid particular emphasis on the social situations in which intergroup conflict occurs.

Realistic Conflict Theory

The various suggestions considered above that intergroup conflict can be seen as the expression of some innate aggressive trait or the aggregation of individual drive states has been the target of sustained criticism from a body of social scientific thinking which Campbell (1965) designated "realistic conflict theory." Identifying a number of common themes in sociology (e.g., Coser, 1956; Sumner, 1906), anthropology (e.g., Leach, 1954), and psychology (e.g., Newcomb, 1960; Sherif, 1966), Campbell suggested that at the heart of this approach was the idea that intergroup behavior can be best understood with reference to the material interests linking groups. Where these are in conflict, rivalry and hostility are thought likely; where they coincide, peace and harmony are the more probable results.

Within social psychology, the most forcible proponent of this view has been Sherif (e.g., 1966) who, in the now classic series of summer camp studies, demonstrated how incompatibility of goals between groups of young boys resulted in intergroup differentiation and antagonism. This hostility was then effectively diminished by the introduction of superordinate goals for the groups. Subsequent research in both field and experimental contexts has largely substantiated Sherif's findings: groups which either adopt or have imposed on them "win-lose" orientations are typically more antagonistic or more discriminatory than those with collaborative orientations (e.g., Blake & Mouton, 1961; Brown, Condor, Mathews, Wade, & Williams, 1985; Brown & Williams, 1984; Diab, 1970; Ryen & Kahn, 1975).

More recently, researchers have begun to suggest some qualifications to the realistic conflict hypothesis (see Turner, 1981a, for a review). For instance, Rabbie and his associates have found important differences between the actual experience of intergroup competition and cooperation and their mere anticipation (e.g., Rabbie & de Brey, 1971; Rabbie & Wilkens, 1971). The general conclusion appears to be that anticipation of competition or cooperation results in weaker effects on intergroup attitudes in the expected directions, provided that at least some degree of ingroup identification has occurred. Where group identification is minimal, differences between anticipated competition and cooperation may disappear (Rabbie & de Brey, 1971). A further problem was identified by Brewer and Campbell (1976) in an ethnographic study of intertribal relations in East Africa. Testing hypotheses developed by LeVine and Campbell (1972) they found positive correlations between socioeconomic similarity, geographical proximity, and attraction for other tribal groups. This was contrary to the realistic conflict hypothesis, since both similarity and proximity should imply increased competition for scarce resources, with resultant intergroup *hostility*. Finally, the imposition of superordinate goals as a recipe for conflict reduction may not always be effective. Blake, Shepard, and Mouton (1964) report instances of organizational conflict which persisted even in the presence of superordinate goals. Indeed, on occasions, superordinate goals may even increase antagonism towards an outgroup. For instance, Worchel, Andreoli, and Folger (1977) found that when intergroup cooperation over common goals was unsuccessful and had been preceded by an episode of competition, liking for the outgroup diminished. Similar results have also been found by Deschamps and Brown (1983) and Brown and Wade (1985), who suggest that intergroup conflict may arise if the cooperative activity results in a lack of task differentiation for the groups concerned.

It therefore appears that functional interdependence per se may not constitute a sufficient predictor of intergroup cooperation. We need to know more about the quality of the intergroup interaction and, relatedly, the nature of the participants' *perceptions* of that interdependence. These are issues to which we shall return later in the chapter (see 'Defining Groups in Social Context,' below).

Social Identity Theory

Other theorists have stressed that intergroup conflict cannot be analyzed in terms of the psychological processes operating in isolated individuals, not only because of the importance of structural intergroup relations, but also because psychological processes may actually be transformed as a result of group membership (e.g., Le Bon, 1897; McDougall, 1919). Although this idea was originally associated with the "group mind" thesis, some theorists who explicitly reject this notion also maintain that group behavior cannot be equated with the behavior of the isolated individual (e.g., Asch 1952).

Of particular contemporary interest is the "intergroup theory" proposed by Tajfel (e.g., 1974), which emphasizes the discontinuities between individuals acting as individuals and acting as members of a group. Whilst Tajfel shares Sherif's concern over structural relations between groups, he also suggests that the discontinuities between individual and group behavior may be attributed to the operation of distinctive psychological processes associated with group membership. This perspective has been greatly elaborated in the social identity (SI) perspective (Tajfel & Turner, 1979; Turner 1982, 1984), which has inspired an enormous amount of research on intergroup relations in recent years (see, e.g., Brown, 1984a; Tajfel, 1978a, 1982b).

The basic assumption of the SI approach is that social categories are employed by individuals not only to simplify their social world (cf. the social cognition approach) but also as a means of self-reference. Categories such as nationality, ethnicity, and gender are internalized and constitute a potentially important aspect of the individual's self-concept, the "social identity" (Turner,

1982; see also Turner's [1984] recent elaboration in terms of "self-categorization theory"). It is suggested that the self is not a static entity, but that when a particular group membership does constitute a salient aspect of the momentary self-image, the individual will come to apply the norms and stereotypes associated with that category to self (Turner, 1982, 1984), and will hence come to regard self as interchangeable with other ingroup members. Through this psychological process (which Turner and his colleagues term "depersonalization"), the individual's behavior becomes normative (conformist), and, to the extent that a number of individuals perceive themselves in terms of the same social category at the same moment in time, collective behavior will occur. Such common self-categorization is not deemed to occur coincidentally, but is regarded as a consequence of the existence of *shared social norms* (Oakes, 1983).

The possibility that an individual's social category membership may constitute an aspect of the *self* concept is seen to have important ramifications for group behavior. Specifically, it is assumed that individuals strive for a satisfactory self-image and that in the course of identifying with a group, this need to perceive oneself positively translates into a need to regard one's group favorably. It is suggested that, since all evaluations of social groups are essentially comparative, the individual does not need only to perceive his or her group positively per se, but rather needs to view the ingroup as "better than" relevant outgroups on appropriate dimensions of comparison (Tajfel, 1978a). Hence, the psychological processes involved in categorization (Doise, 1978) and a motivation for positive self-evaluation (Turner, 1975) lead to a situation in which individuals to whom group membership is salient will seek to differentiate ingroup from outgroup on valued dimensions. It is, however, stressed that this competitive orientation need not imply that intergroup relations will always be characterized by overt conflict (Turner, 1981a), and it is an important issue for future research to investigate when it is that this competitive potential is actually manifested in a hostile form.

The SI perspective has been closely associated with research conducted in the so-called minimal group paradigm (MGP), in which subjects are divided into groups on trivial or even explicitly random criteria, having no knowledge of, or communication with, other in- and outgroup members and there being no "realistic" conflict of interest between the groups. It has been quite reliably found that in such situations individuals will distribute monetary rewards or meaningless points in such a way as to maximize the relative superiority of ingroup over outgroup, even if this involves a forfeit in absolute ingroup gain (see Brewer, 1979; Turner, 1978). In emphasizing the importance of comparative rather than absolute evaluation in intergroup conflict, the SI approach is consistent with other perspectives which have emphasized the need to maintain differentials as a motivating force in gaming situations (Tropper, 1972) and as a frustrating trigger for aggression (Feierabend & Feierabend, 1966).

A particular area of concern to SI theorists has been the way in which the need for positive social identity may influence the behavior of low status social groups (e.g., Brown, 1978; Caddick, 1982; Commins & Lockwood, 1979; Skevington, 1981; Tajfel, 1978b). In this the SI model has an obvious advantage over earlier perspectives which attempted to attribute conflict initiated by ruling groups to different psychological mechanisms from that initiated by subordinate groups: for example, accounting for intranational unrest in terms of irrationality and international conflict as an unfortunate error of rational processes (see Billig, 1976).

Although SI theorists have strongly emphasized the distinction between their approach and previous social psychological formulations of intergroup conflict, it appears that the literature can only benefit from a closer association between the SI perspective and other social psychological approaches (Condor, Williams, & Brown, 1984). For example, the adoption of an SI perspective need not preclude a concern for individual differences in predisposition to hostile intergroup activity. Research suggests that individuals may differ in their thresholds for perceiving groups as entities (see Horwitz & Rabbie, 1982) and that differences in self-consciousness may affect an individual's propensity to identify with a social group (Abrams, 1984). Downing and Monaco (1979) suggest that levels of ingroup favoritism displayed in minimal group settings may be influenced by authoritarianism, and Billig (1978) also notes the utility of this concept in his intergroup approach to Fascism. However, it is notable that in minimal (Brown, Tajfel, & Turner, 1980) and more "realistic" (Condor et al., 1984) settings the behavior of group members may be determined more by situational factors influencing the salience of group membership than preexisting "individual differences." This is, of course, consistent with field studies of ethnic prejudice which demonstrate that individual differences may explain variation in prejudicial attitudes within rather than between particular social contexts (Pettigrew, 1958).

Applying Psychological Theories of Intergroup Conflict

It is now well recognised that psychological functioning and activity always take place in a social context, such that even laboratory experiments should be regarded as constituting a particular (albeit rather atypical) form of social situation (e.g., Tajfel, 1980; Turner, 1981b). Since no behavior operates in a "social vacuum" (Tajfel, 1972), psychological theories concerning intergroup conflict in abstract need to be supplemented by an understanding of the *particular* manifestation of actual instances of conflictual relations between social groups. In the following pages we will outline some of the considerations necessary to apply abstract psychological theories to actual instances of intergroup conflict as it occurs not only in the field, but also in the "controlled" experimental laboratory.

Defining Groups in Social Context

The fundamental problem in analyzing intergroup conflict is that of postulating the existence of social groups. This is, of course, often not an issue in the laboratory, where certain systems of social categorization may be defined and imposed by the experimenter. With respect to naturalistic groups, SI theorists have emphasized the need to define group membership subjectively rather than relying on the perspective of the researcher as external observer (Tajfel, 1978a; Turner, 1982). However, the tendency towards objectification continues. For example, researchers have assumed a priori that women constitute a social group (Kalmuss, Gurin, & Townsend, 1981; Williams & Giles, 1978; but cf. Breakwell, 1979; Condor, 1983). Whether people actually *do* act in terms of any particular social category is, of course, a matter for empirical investigation rather than a priori assumption (see also Parkin, 1971; Westergaard, 1975, for a discussion of this issue with respect to social class).

The suggestion by SI researchers that the existence of social groups should be sought in the subjectivity of the actors naturally raises the important question of *whose* subjectivity is considered in particular situations of intergroup conflict. It is, of course, possible that only one party may recognize the existence of an ingroup-outgroup distinction (see, e.g., Deschamps, 1982). Moreover, it may be the case that within a single conflictual situation actors sharing a common social identification may nonetheless hold different perceptions concerning their protagonist. For instance, members of the Greenham Common women's peace camp variously characterize themselves as opposing men, capitalism, the British police, and the American military. When applying their perspectives to naturalistic conflict, social psychologists should set *as their first task* an analysis of the presence and limits of social groups and the relationship between them.

An application of general theories to particular instances of intergroup conflict demands a consideration not only of the existence but also of the meaning of social groups. The suggestion that the results of laboratory studies may be generalized in terms of process rather than manifestation (Turner, 1981b) may lead some to the dangerous assumption that the specific characteristics of particular groups are unimportant. Individual differences theorists such as Adorno and colleagues focus their attention on prejudice per se, rather than on any particular manifestation of intergroup conflict (see Billig, 1976). Similarly, concern for process leads SI theorists to formulate general, abstract rules concerning such factors as perceived similarity between groups (Brown, 1984b; Turner, 1978) and the tendency to differentiate ingroup from outgroup (Tajfel & Turner, 1979). However, the fact that minimal group research has demonstrated that groups may engage in ingroup favoritism in terms of "meaningless points" does not obviate the need to consider which ingroup-outgroup distinctions are emphasized in a particular situation of intergroup conflict. Although it appears fairly self-evident that an understanding of any particular instance of social conflict would involve an analysis of the way in which intergroup relations are ideologically represented, several attempts have been made to conduct research which is apparently based on the assumption that all social categories may be regarded as interchangeable. For example, Doise et al. (1978) and van Knippenberg, Pruyn, & Wilke (1982) report studies using males and females to test abstract hypotheses concerning the accentuation of intercategory differences in collective encounters, only to be forced to consider the *particular* sociological and ideological aspects of the sex category system in order to provide a post hoc interpretation of their data.

The problem is not confined to the mere identification of particular characteristics associated with in- and outgroup (what Ashmore & Del Boca, 1981, term the "cataloging" approach to stereotyping). It is also important to understand the symbolic significance of these particular stereotyped attributes in the particular intergroup context in which they are used. For example, where social hierarchies are regarded as achieved rather than ascribed, it is important for dominant social groups to stress their intellectual superiority over the dominated (Perkins, 1979). Hence, "similarities" and "differences" between groups cannot be fully understood without an appreciation of their possible symbolic significance in the search for material advantage (see, e.g., Condor, 1985; Hewstone & Jaspars, 1984; van Knippenberg, 1984).

The importance of "realistic" dimensions of intergroup conflict is still largely overlooked even in post-Sherifian social psychological analyses. Notwithstanding the validity of Turner's (1975) distinction between "realistic" and "social" conflict, it remains the case that in naturalistic settings intergroup conflict may become associated with material conflicts of interest even if these do not represent the original cause of the antagonism (see, e.g., Tajfel, 1977). When psychologists do consider material conflicts of interest they are often tempted to merely document material inequalities which may be observed objectively (e.g., Capozza, Bonaldo, & DiMaggio, 1982; Jaspars & Warnaen, 1982; Williams & Giles, 1978). However, as Tajfel & Turner (1979) emphasize, it is *perceived* rather than "objective" conflicts of interest which are likely to be important in directing intergroup activity. For example, many researchers have assumed that members of objectively defined minority groups will experience a low sense of self-worth (e.g., Cartwright, 1950). Such perspectives overlook the possibility of "false consciousness," which may obscure the existence of intergroup status differentials from minority groups (Gramsci, 1971) and hence protect the identity of group members (Condor & Abrams, 1984).

In order to understand the ideological representation of social groups within particular conflictual settings, it is essential to adopt an historical perspective. The social psychological experimentalist may fail to develop the habit of regarding intergroup conflict historically (cf. Kelvin, 1984), since in the typical laboratory intergroup imagery and behavior have no past and no future beyond the immediate experimental context. For example, researchers often regard stereotyping as the processing of preexisting information rather than as the creation of strategic intergroup imagery (e.g., Eagly & Steffen, 1984). An appreciation of history would, by contrast, emphasize how both traditional and revolutionary social imagery may also be regarded as future-directed, aimed at maintaining or changing social reality, rather than as a passive recognition of existing conditions (Bourhis & Hill, 1982; see also Sherif, 1966).

A consideration of goal orientation in particular instances of intergroup conflict may, however, lead to problems for statements of psychological theory concerning intergroup conflict *in general.* While some approaches (notably F-A theory) merely postulate the observable effects of prior physical or social conditions, the suggestion that social conflict arises from a prior "need" for hostility (e.g., Simmel, 1955), or that individuals use social categories *in order to* simplify their social world (Hamilton, 1981) are obviously teleogical. Despite the advantage of Tajfel's (1981b) analysis of social stereotyping in social context, this is problematic in its tendency to infer the manifest functions of existing stereotypes from an observation of existing social conditions. The functionalism inherent in the suggestion that intergroup imagery exists in order to "create" intergroup inequality might, of course, be avoided by focusing on the way in which particular stereotypes are used in social rhetoric aimed at maintaining or changing the status quo.

Power Relations in Intergroup Conflict

We have argued that in applying general social psychological theory to actual instances of intergroup conflict it is essential to understand the way in which social groups are represented subjectively. However, in itself this is inadequate without a simultaneous appreciation of the way in which power is distributed in a particular intergroup setting. The issue of power is typically overlooked by intergroup researchers (Apfelbaum, 1979); for example, experimental analogies (as in gaming research) or actual instances of intergroup conflict (e.g., Sherif, 1966) tend to be created without power distinctions between subjects. The issue of power is obviously important in determining how groups are defined (Deschamps, 1982; Gallagher, 1983), the stereotypes associated with them (e.g. van Knippenberg, 1978), and the ability to transform subjective ingroup favoritism into action (Ng, 1982). Although SI theorists have often considered the issue of power relations in an abstract sense, this is rarely followed through in their theorizing or research. For example, Tajfel's (1981b) discussion of the "social functions" of social stereotypes concentrates on the issues of what functions stereotypes may serve for groups at the expense of the equally important question of *for whom* they serve these functions, and research within the MGP has typically overlooked the importance of power relations between groups (Ng, 1982). The fact that psychologists are able to construct instances of intergroup conflict characterized by equal power between the protagonists cannot be taken to suggest that power is unimportant even in the laboratory, since the very presence of intergroup conflict (or harmony) is a reflection of the power of the experimenter to create social categories and influence the distribution of resources and channels of communication between them (Billig, 1976).

A consideration of the question of power is particularly important if we are to attempt to apply psychological premises to the resolution of social conflict. For example, analyses of intergroup conflict in the abstract may lead us to suggest that superordinate goals will lead to conflict resolution (Sherif, 1966). The problem is that it is likely that these superordinate goals will, themselves, be formulated within the context of the intergroup conflict which they aim to resolve: witness, for example, the subordination of the interests of minority groups to the "superordinate" goal of national unity. Indeed, it is evidently the case that in Sherif's own field studies the imposition of superordinate goals was implemented by, and served the purposes of, a particular powerful group – the experimenters (Billig, 1976). In the same way, the suggestion that intergroup conflict may be resolved by the creation of complementary group distinctiveness (e.g., Taylor & Simard, 1977; Turner, 1981b) cannot be implemented without an acknowledgement of the power relations between social groups existing in any particular naturalistic intergroup setting. Indeed, social representations of intergroup "complementarity" (e.g., of the sexes) and symbiosis (e.g., of management and workforce) represent one of the most powerful ideological weapons used to *maintain* inequitable intergroup relations.

Although we have argued for a need to define groups and their meaning subjectively, there does appear to be a case for social psychologists to consider power relations as an *objective* aspect of the social world. It is possible for power relationships to affect social cognition and activity without the awareness of the group members involved (e.g., Henley, 1977). It is for this reason that ascendant minority groups often emphasize the need for "consciousness raising."

The tendency to overlook the importance of social ideology and power in the relations between social groups is not simply naive. To the extent that social psychologists adopt a social problem approach to this field, it is also potentially dangerous. Billig (1976, p.120) notes how an overemphasis on the psychological rather than the social-structural determinants of intergroup conflict may restrict efforts directed toward social change: "People may not be able to undo their own childhoods, but they are able to change collectively the nature of their society."

Thus far we have emphasized the obvious difficulties involved in contextualizing general psychological theories such that they are relevant to particular instances of intergroup conflict. We will now turn to consider a problem associated with the relationship between research, theory, and application. Specifically, we will be suggesting that an uncritical reliance on *experimental* methodology – whether conducted in the laboratory or the field – may lead us to inadvertently adopt a particular "model of man" which may restrict our understanding of the interplay between psychological and social factors in particular situations of intergroup conflict.

Psychological Process and Social Context

We have already noted Turner's (1981b) suggestion that laboratory research may be applicable to the "real world" in terms of underlying processes rather than particular empirical manifestations of psychological functioning. One problem which Turner does not solve is that of identifying what is process (and therefore generalizable) and what is manifestation (and therefore peculiar to the particular context in which it is observed). The classic experimental model presupposes such prior knowledge, leading us to represent events in terms of simple causal sequences: "stimulus" and "response," "cause" and "effect"; or, to use Turner's (1981b) own example, we talk about X "producing" Y. It is easy to see how the transposition of methodological logic into statements of theory may lead to necessarily futile chicken-and-egg arguments concerning psychological priority in intergroup conflict.

The problem of postulating any phenomena as "basic" to social behavior is most clearly apparent in theories which imply that the psychological roots of intergroup conflict such as aggressive drives or color prejudice may be reduced to still more "basic" biological factors (e.g., Lorenz, 1967; Williams & Morland, 1976). Although the individual differences approaches to intergroup conflict were originally developed in order to avoid biological reductionism, they face problems associated with postulating *psychological* primacy. Take, for example, the tenuous distinction draw between (prior) "personality" and (emergent) "attitude" (e.g., Adorno et al., 1950; Eysenck & Wilson, 1978; Rokeach, 1960). The proposition that authoritarian/dogmatic attitudes are expressed by authoritarian or dogmatic personalities is obviously tautologous and becomes particularly problematic when it is considered that attempts to measure ("fundamental") personality typically utilize indices of ("emergent") attitude.

Similar problems are involved in theoretical statements formulated on the basis of the MGP, in which categorization is treated as an independent variable, which when manipulated may *result in* group conflict (Brown et al., 1980). Although it is obviously important to demonstrate that intergroup conflict may arise in the absence of material conflicts of interest, extending this empirical observation to general theoretical statements threatens to substitute one hypothesized absolute causal factor (realistic conflict) for another (social categorization/comparison). For example, Turner and Giles (1981, p. 26) suggest that "categorization and social comparison processes are complementary determinants [sic] of intergroup discrimination." In the "real" social psychological world cause-and-effect cannot be so carefully demarcated, and postulating causal sequences merely begs the question of what causes the "basic" phenomena in the sequence; we might reasonably ask what causes the social categorization which Turner and Giles suggest leads to intergroup discrimination. Simple statements of cause-and-effect belie the subtlety of the SI approach which recognizes the problems of postulating essential priority for any particular psychological process. Thus, social categorization can be regarded as both dependent on and itself enhancing perceived intragroup similarity (e.g., Turner, 1984). Similarly, phenomena such as self-esteem (see Abrams & Hogg, 1984) and social conflict (Brown & Turner, 1981) can be represented as both dependent and independent variables in intergroup relations. This, however, leads to a paradox in that when social psychologists do characterize psychological functioning as a feedback system this conflicts with the demands of experimental methodology for formal, testable (often directional) theory, and can hence lead to tautology.[1]

Problems do not only arise in attempting to identify "basic" psychological processes in intergroup conflict. If these psychological processes are to be regarded as a feedback system, so must this system be regarded as "open" to social context. Sherif's (1966, p. 2) opposition to attempts to analyze intergroup conflict in terms of "human nature in the raw" is shared by many personality theorists (e. g., Sanford, 1973) and by intergroup researchers who emphasize how "the social setting of intergroup relations contributes to making ... individuals what they are and they in turn produce this social setting: they and it develop symbiotically" (Tajfel, 1972, p. 95). At the same time, social psychologists often imply that some aspects of psychological functioning may be regarded as "basic" to social behavior. For example, SI researchers typically regard social identification and intergroup differentiation as universal processes which may simply vary in their manifestation (see Wetherell, 1982; Williams, 1984, for criticisms of this approach).

There is a corresponding problem in the obverse tendency to regard sociological phenomena as somehow fundamental and preexistent to human psychology and activity. Psychologists often allude to the influence of "wider social factors" such as economics or social norms in situations of intergroup conflict (e. g., Berkowitz, 1962; Roheim, 1950), but exclude these from their own analyses, deeming them to be the proper province of the historian, sociologist, economist, or anthropologist. However, social psychologists are doing their discipline a disservice if they fail to recognize that "social" phenomena necessarily arise from, and are maintained by, human cognition and motivation. The idea that social phenomena may be regarded as simply imposed upon preexisting individuals is common in the social psychological literature (see, e. g., Tajfel, 1972), and is probably exacerbated by the reluctance of researchers to recognize their own role as causal agent in experimental contexts.

The tendency to divorce social context from psychological processes is well illustrated by approaches to intergroup imagery which regard preexisting "similarities" and "differences" to be imposed upon the individual's perception of social groups. For example, Nye (1973, p. 34) informs us that "social pressure is a potent force that often impels individuals to become prejudiced," and the authors of the Authoritarian Personality (Adorno et al. 1950) regard cultural stereotypes and social categories as preexisting, ready for the individual to pluck if

---

1 As a further example we may cite SI theorists' a priori definition of group membership in terms of self-categorization (Turner's [1981a] "social identification model"). The argument is then transformed to suggest that social identification *determines* group formation: "Individuals may become a group simply because they perceive themselves to share some form of discontinuous homogeneity" (Turner, 1981a, p. 90), and behavior (Turner's [1981a] "social identity principle"): "The consequences of depersonalization are ... the various phenomena of group behaviour" (Turner, 1984, p. 35). To some extent, this objection should be regarded as pedantic. However, it is worth bearing in mind that Tajfel originally opted for an explanation of intergroup discrimination in terms of intrapsychic processes on the basis that alternative explanations in terms of generic social norms were both circular and nonheuristic!

so disposed. Whilst it is doubtless true that social representations may preexist the individual social perceiver, we should not overlook the fact that stereotypes and the categories with which they are associated represent social psychological *constructions* (Berger & Luckmann, 1967; Tajfel, 1981 a, b; Turner, 1984). Various authors have documented the way in which such apparently "natural" categories such as sex (Kessler & McKenna 1978) and race (Miles, 1982; Reicher, 1986) have actually been *created* and how their form is bound up with the intergroup conflict of which they are a part.

The habit of regarding social forces as existing outside of human psychological functioning is not restricted to analyses of social ideology, but also to aspects of the intergroup "infrastructure" [sic]. Again, this appears in part an intellectual legacy of the experimental technique of imposing social structural arrangements upon the "basic psychological processes" of a collection of "subjects" in the traditional laboratory experimental setting (e. g., Turner & Brown, 1978). It is, of course, the case that even in the experiment these status differences are created by human activity: that of the experimenter. However, overlooking this fact may lead to generalized statements which attempt to contextualize psychological theories of social conflict without due regard for human agency. The authoritarian personality authors suggest that "People are continuously moulded from above because they must be moulded if the over-all economic pattern is to be maintained ..." (Adorno et al., 1950, p. 976). In some mystical way the disembodied economic context in the naturalistic environment takes on the role of E in the laboratory. More recently, we have seen theories which imply that contact is something which is imposed on social groups, rather than a solution developed *by* them (Hewstone & Brown, 1986). Attempts to socialize the F-A hypothesis by postulating that frustration may be engendered by "aversive" social events such as economic privation (Konečni, 1979) leave open the question of where these "aversive events" originate from, if not from the activity of human beings. Similarly, Sherif's (1966) boys camp studies leave us with the feeling that "conflicts of interest" and "superordinate goals" are somehow thrust upon groups by some unexplained external force. However, if social psychological theories are to have any applied relevance, such a conceptual splitting off of psychological processes from social context is potentially dangerous. To overlook the fact that zero-sum games are *created* (by E) can easily encourage the conclusion that the social preconditions for the arms race have been imposed on rational individuals by mystical alien forces rather than arising from, and only likely to be changed by, human action.

Concluding Comments

Our aim in this chapter has been a modest one. We have not attempted to provide a comprehensive analysis of psychological work on intergroup conflict, and we are only too aware of having excluded some important issues in our whirlwind tour. For example, we have not considered the possible effect of intergroup conflict on individual psychology (e. g., Gillespie, 1942), nor the way in which psychological theories and research may themselves represent a part of the very situations of intergroup conflict which they seek to explain (see, e.g., Billig, 1982). Our concern has been limited to the explication of some of the problems inherent in the interrelationship between psychological theory, research, and application. We may extract a number of themes raised in the preceding pages which may serve as conlusions.

1. Many psychological theories have attempted to explain intergroup conflict either in terms of "normal" drives or in terms of "normal" cognitive functioning. There is a need for further integration of these two areas, in particular an analysis of how "normal" motivation may be related to the "normal" cognitive functioning associated with categorization and stereotyping.

2. Intergroup conflict is, by definition, a collective phenomenon, and requires a suitably collective "model of man." The psychological factors associated with intergroup hostility are best sought in *collective* social cognition and motivation. It is an important task for the social psychologist to examine the relationship between individual drives and cognition and those associated with the groups to which they belong; for example, the relationship between individual racism and national immigration laws (see Milner, 1981).

3. In analyzing the psychological aspects of intergroup conflict we should be aware that motivational and cognitive processes necessarily operate in a social context. This is, of course, highlighted when applying psychological perspectives on intergroup conflict to the field, where it becomes apparent that a direct application of laboratory findings may result in not so much an incomplete as a spurious picture of specific instances of intergroup conflict. After all, if psychological functioning in intergroup conflict were not affected by social context, there would be no need for "controlled" laboratory studies in the first place!

4. Most field researchers pay lip service to the need to contextualize psychological theories, but this cannot be done by simply observing sociological phenomena rather than understanding the way in which these are represented in social ideology and hence the consciousness of social actors. In particular, a full understanding of intergroup conflict needs to take account of the way in which ingroup-outgroup imagery becomes associated symbolically with realistic intergroup conflict. Moreover, as Sherif (1966, p. 21) emphasized, "The psychology of intergroup attitudes and behavior must specify contemporary events within the framework of the past relationships between people and their future goals and designs." We would add that such an approach must also be sensitive to the power available to social groups to define and to act upon particular situations of intergroup conflict.

5. One factor which threatens the applicability of psychological approaches to intergroup conflict is the tendency for methodological considerations to infiltrate abstract theory. The major danger in this respect appears to be the "independent variable," which emerges in our theorizing in terms of postulates concerning which psychological process may "cause" another, and whether intergroup conflict may be "basically" attributed to biology, psychology, or society. "Independent" variables simply *do not exist* in the real world, and the as-

sumption that they do will not only cause our theory to stagnate, but also limit our understanding of intergroup conflict as it occurs in the laboratory. Rather than methodology influencing theory, it should be the case that psychological theory (acknowledging the dialectical nature of psychological and social functioning) aids our interpretation of laboratory experimentation such that we recognize that so-called independent variables are actually dependent on the intervention of E.

6. In attempting to contextualize psychological theories of intergroup conflict it is essential that psychology and society be regarded as inextricably *inter*dependent. We cannot postulate psychology as somehow ontologically prior to the social contexts in which it is manifested; reification of social events into psychological processes effectively prevents the development of dynamic theory capable of accounting for social change (Reicher, 1984). However, by the same token, we reject entirely the claim that intergroup conflict can be understood without recourse to psychological processes (cf. Dahrendorf, 1958). Wars, as the UNESCO charter states, obviously begin in the minds of men [sic]. This suggestion is only reductionistic to the extent that we employ an individualistic, asocial model of human psychology. Social groups are made by people, and antagonism caused by people. To overlook this most self-evident of social psychological truths is to deny human responsibility for intergroup conflict.

References

Abrams, D. (1984). *Social identity, self consciousness and intergroup behaviour.* Unpublished doctoral thesis, University of Kent, Canterbury.

Abrams, D., & Hogg, M. A. (1984, July). *Social identity, self-esteem and intergroup discrimination: a critical re-examination.* Paper presented at the Annual Conference of the British Psychological Society (Social Psychology Section), Oxford.

Adorno, T. W., Frenkel-Brunswick, E., Levinson, D. J., & Sanford, R. N. (1950). *The Authoritarian Personality.* New York: Harper & Row.

Allport, G. W. (1954). *The Nature of Prejudice.* Cambridge, MA: Addison-Wesley.

Apfelbaum, E. (1979). Relations of domination and movements for liberation: an analysis of power between groups. W. Austin & S. Worchel (Eds.), *The Social Psychology of Intergroup Relations.* Monterey, CA: Brooks/Cole.

Asch, S. E. (1952). *Social Psychology.* Englewood Cliffs, NJ: Prentice-Hall.

Ashmore, R. D., & Del Boca, F. K. (1976). Psychological approaches to understanding intergroup conflicts. In P. A. Katz (Ed.), *Towards the Elimination of Racism.* New York: Pergamon.

Ashmore, R. D., & Del Boca, F. K. (1979). Sex stereotypes and implicit personality theory: Toward a cognitive-social psychological conceptualization. *Sex Roles, 6,* 501–18.

Ashmore, R. D., & Del Boca, F. K. (1981) Conceptual approaches to stereotypes and stereotyping. In D. L. Hamilton (Ed.), *Cognitive processes in stereotyping and intergroup behavior.* Hillsdale, NJ: Erlbaum.

Ashmore, R. D., & Tumia, M. (1980). Sex stereotypes and implicit personality theory 1: A personality description approach to the assessment of sex stereotypes. *Sex Roles, 6,* 501–18.

Bem, S. L. (1981). Gender schema theory: A cognitive account of sex typing. *Psychological Review, 88,* 356–364.

Berger, P. L., & Luckmann, T. (1967). *The social construction of reality.* London: Allen Lane.

Berkowitz, L. (1962). *Aggression: A social psychological analysis.* New York: McGraw-Hill.

Berkowitz, L. (1969). The frustration-aggression hypothesis revisited. In L. Berkowitz (Ed.), *Roots of aggression.* New York: Atherton.

Billig, M. (1976). *Social psychology and intergroup relations.* London: Academic.

Billig, M. (1978). *Fascists: A social psychological view of the national front.* London: Academic.

Billig, M. (1982). *Ideology and social psychology.* Oxford: Blackwell.

Billig, M. (1985). Prejudice, categorisation and particularisation: From a perceptual to a rhetorical approach. *European Journal of Social Psychology, 15,* 79–103.

Blake, R. R., & Mouton, J. S. (1961). *Group dynamics: key to decision-making.* Houston: Gulf.

Blake, R. R., Shepard, H. A., & Mouton, J. S. (1964). *Managing intergroup conflict in industry.* Houston: Gulf.

Bourhis, R. Y., & Hill, P. (1982). Intergroup perceptions in British higher education: A field study. In H. Tajfel (Ed.), *Social identity and intergroup relations.* Cambridge & Paris: Cambridge University Press and Editions de la Maison des Sciences de l'Homme.

Breakwell, G. (1979). Woman: Group and identity? *Women's Studies International Quarterly, 2,* 9–17.

Brewer, M. B. (1979). Ingroup bias in the minimal group situation: A cognitive-motivational analysis. *Psychological Bulletin, 86,* 307–324.

Brewer, M. B., & Campbell, D. T. (1976). *Ethnocentrism and intergroup attitudes: East African evidence.* New York: Sage.

Brewer, M. B., & Kramer, R. M. (1985). The psychology of intergroup attitudes and behavior. *Annual Review of Psychology, 36,* 219–243.

Brown, R. (1965). *Social psychology.* New York: MacMillan.

Brown, R. J. (1978). Divided we fall: An analysis of relations between sections of a factory workforce. In H. Tajfel (Ed.), *Differentiation between social groups: Studies in the social psychology of intergroup relations.* London: Academic.

Brown, R. J. (1984 a). *British Journal of Social Psychology, 23,* Special Issue on Intergroup Processes.

Brown, R. J. (1984 b). The effects of intergroup similarity and cooperative vs competitive orientation on intergroup discrimination. *British Journal of Social Psychology, 23,* 21–33.

Brown, R. J., Condor, S., Mathews, A., Wade, G., & Williams, J. (1985). Explaining intergroup differentiation in organisations. Unpublished manuscript, University of Kent, Canterbury.

Brown, R. J., Tajfel, H., & Turner, J. C. (1980). Minimal group situation and intergroup discrimination: Comment on the paper by Aschenbrenner and Schafer. *European Journal of Social Psychology, 10,* 399–414.

Brown, R. J., & Turner, J. C. (1981). Interpersonal and intergroup behaviour. In J. C. Turner & H. Giles (Eds.), *Intergroup behaviour.* Oxford: Blackwell.

Brown, R. J., & Wade, G. (1985) Superordinate goals and intergroup behaviour: The effects of role ambiguity on intergroup attitudes and task performance. Unpublished manuscript, University of Kent, Canterbury.

Brown, R. J., & Williams, J. (1984). Group identifications: The same thing to all people? *Human Relations, 37,* 547–564.

Caddick, B. (1982). Perceived illegitimacy and intergroup relations. In H. Tajfel (Ed.), *Social identity and intergroup relations.* Cambridge & Paris: Cambridge University Press & Editions de la Maison des Sciences de l'Homme.

Campbell, D. T. (1965). Ethnocentric and other altruistic motives. In D. Levine (Ed.) *Nebraska Symposium on Motivation* (Vol. 13). Lincoln: University of Nebraska Press.

Capozza, D., Bonaldo, E., & DiMaggio, A. (1982). Problems of identity and social conflict: Research on ethnic groups in Italy. In H. Tajfel (Ed.), *Social identity and intergroup relations.* Cambridge & Paris: Cambridge University Press and Editions de la Maison des Sciences de l'Homme.

Cartwright, D. (1950). Emotional dimensions of group life. In M. L. Reymert (Ed.), *International symposium on feelings and emotions.* New York: McGraw-Hill.

Cherniss, C. (1972). Personality and ideology: A personological study of women's liberation. *Psychiatry, 35,* 109–125.

Cherry, F., & Byrne, D. (1977). Authoritarianism. In T. Blass (Ed.), *Personality variables in social behavior.* Hillsdale, NJ: Erlbaum.

Christie, R., & Jahoda, M. (Eds.) (1954). *Studies in the scope and method of the authoritarian personality*. New York: Free Press.

Commins, B., & Lockwood, J. (1979). The effects of status differences, favored treatment and equity on intergroup comparisons. *European Journal of Social Psychology, 9,* 281-289.

Condor, S. (1983, December). *Conceptualising women as a social group*. Paper presented at the British Psychological Association Conference, London.

Condor, S. (1985). *Womanhood as an aspect of social identity*. Unpublished doctoral thesis, University of Bristol.

Condor, S., & Abrams, D. (1984, July). *Womanhood as an aspect of social identity: group identification and ideology*. Paper presented at the British Psychological Society's International Conference on Self and Identity, University College Cardiff, Wales.

Condor, S., Williams, J., & Brown, R.J. (1984, July). *Identity, intragroup relations and intergroup behaviour*. Paper presented at the British Psychological Society (Social Psychology Section) Annual Conference, Oxford.

Coser, L. (1956). *Functions of social conflict*. New York: Free Press.

Crawford, T.J., & Nadich, M. (1970). Relative deprivation, powerlessness and militance: The psychology of social protest. *Psychiatry, 33,* 208-223.

Dahrendorf, R. (1958). Toward a theory of social conflict. *Journal of Conflict Resolution, 2,* 170-183.

Davies, J.C. (1973). Aggression, violence, revolution, and war. In J.N.Knutson (Ed.), *Handbook of political psychology*. San Francisco: Jossey-Bass.

Davis, D.R. (1963). The psychological mechanisms of maladaptive behaviour. In M.Penrose (Ed.), *Pathogenesis of war*. London: Lewis.

Deschamps, J.C. (1982). Social identity and relations of power between groups. In H.Tajfel (Ed.), *Social identity and intergroup relations*. Cambridge & Paris: Cambridge University Press and Editions de la Maison des Sciences de l'Homme.

Deschamps, J.-C., & Brown, R.J. (1983). Superordinate goals and intergroup conflict. *British Journal of Social Psychology, 22,* 189-195.

Deutsch, M. (1973). *The resolution of conflict*. London: Yale University Press.

Diab, L. (1970). A study of intragroup and intergroup relations among experimentally produced small groups. *Genetic Psychology Monographs, 82,* 49-82.

Dicks, H.V. (1950). Personality traits and national socialist ideology. *Human Relations, 3,* 111-154.

Doise, W. (1978). *Groups and individuals: Explanations in social psychology*. Cambridge: Cambridge University Press.

Doise, W., Deschamps, J.-C., & Meyer, G. (1978). The accentuation of intracategory similarities. In H.Tajfel (Ed.), *Differentiation between social groups: Studies in the social psychology of intergroup relations*. London: Academic.

Dollard, J., Miller, N.E., Doob, L.W., Mowrer, O.H., & Sears, R.R. (1939). *Frustration and aggression*. New Haven: Yale University Press.

Downing, L.L., & Monaco, N.R. (1979). *Ingroup-outgroup bias formation as a function of differential ingroup-outgroup contact and authoritarian personality: A field experiment*. Mimeo, Union College, Schenectady.

Durbin, E.F.M., & Bowlby, J. (1938). *Personal aggressiveness and war*. London: Routledge & Kegan Paul.

Eagly, A., & Steffen, V. (1984). Gender stereotypes stem from the distribution of men and women into social roles. *Journal of Personality and Social Psychology, 46,* 735-754.

Eiser, J.R. (1980). *Cognitive social psychology*. London: McGraw-Hill.

Etzioni, A. (1969). Social-psychological aspects of international relations. In G.Lindsay & E.Aronson (Eds.), *The handbook of social psychology: Vol.5. Applied social psychology* (2nd ed). Reading, MA: Addison-Wesley.

Eysenck, H., & Wilson, G. (1978). *The psychological basis of ideology*. Lancaster: MTP Press.

Feierabend, I.K., & Feierabend, R.L. (1966). Aggressive behavior within political violence: Cross-national patterns. In H.D.Graham & T.R.Gurr (Eds.), *Violence in america*. New York: Bantam.

Fiedler, F.E. (1967). *A theory of leadership effectiveness*. New York: McGraw-Hill.

Forward, J.R., & Williams, J.R. (1970). Internal-external locus of control and black militancy. *Journal of Social issues, 26,* 75-92.

Freud, S. (1961). *Group psychology and the analysis of the ego. In J. Strachey (Ed. and Trans.) The standard edition of the complete psychological works.* London: Hogarth. (Original work published 1921).

Fromm, E. (1977. *The anatomy of human destructiveness.* Harmondsworth: Penguin.

Gallagher, A. (1983). *Ideology and social conflict.* Paper presented at the Sixth Annual Scientific Meeting of the International Society of Political Psychology.

Gardner, R.C. (1973). Ethnic stereotypes: The traditional approach: A new look. *The Canadian Psychologist, 14,* 133-148.

Gillespie, M.D. (1942). *Psychological effects of war on citizen and soldier.* New York: Norton.

Gramsci, A. (1971). *Selections from the prison notebooks.* (Q. Hoare & G. Nowell-Smith, Eds. and Trans.). London: Lawrence & Wishart.

Hamilton, D.L. (Ed.). (1981). *Cognitive processes in stereotyping and intergroup behavior.* Hillsdale, NJ: Erlbaum.

Henley, N. (1977). *Body politics.* Englewood Cliffs, NJ: Prentice-Hall.

Herman, M.G., & Herman, C.F. (1982). A look inside the 'black box': Building on a decade of research. In G. Hopple (Ed.), *Biopolitics, political psychology and international politics.* London, Frances Pinter.

Hewstone, M., & Brown, R.J. (1986). *Contact and conflict in intergroup encounters.* Oxford: Blackwell.

Hewstone, M., & Jaspars, J. (1984). Social dimensions of attribution. In H. Tajfel (Ed.), *The social dimension: European developments in social psychology* (Vol. 2). Cambridge & Paris: Cambridge University Press & Editions de la Maison des Sciences de l'Homme.

Himmelweit, H. (1950). Frustration and aggression: A review of recent experimental work. In T.H. Pear (Ed.), *Psychological factors of peace and war.* London & New York: Hutchinson.

Hollander, E.D. (1978). *Leadership dynamics: A practical guide to effective relationships.* New York: Free Press.

Horwitz, M., & Rabbie, J.M. (1982). Individuality and membership in the intergroup system. In H. Tajfel (Ed.), *Social identity and intergroup relations.* Cambridge & Paris: Cambridge University Press and Editions de la Maison des Sciences de l'Homme.

Jaspars, J., & Warnaen, S. (1982). Intergroup relations, ethnic identity and self-evaluation in Indonesia. In H. Tajfel (Ed.), *Social identity and intergroup relations.* Cambridge & Paris: Cambridge University Press and Editions de la Maison des Sciences de l'Homme.

Kalmuss, D., Gurin, D., & Townsend, A. (1981). Feminist and sympathetic feminist consciousness. *European Journal of Social Psychology, 11,* 131-147.

Katz, D. (1961). Current and needed psychological research in international relations. *Journal of Social Issues, 17,* 69-78.

Katz, D., & Braly, K. (1933). Social stereotypes of one hundred college students. *Journal of Abnormal and Social Psychology, 28,* 280-290.

Kelley, H.H. (1968). Interpersonal accommodation. *American Psychologist, 23,* 399-410.

Kelvin, P. (1984). The historical dimension of social psychology: the case of unemployment. In H. Tajfel (Ed.), *The social dimension: European developments in social psychology* (Vol. 2). Cambridge and Paris: Cambridge University Press & Editions de la Maison des Sciences de l'Homme.

Kessler, S.J., & McKenna, W. (1978). *Gender: An ethnomethodological approach.* New York: Wiley-Interscience.

Kirsch, J.P., & Dillehay, R.C. (1967). *Dimensions of authoritarianism.* University of Kentucky Press.

Klineberg, O. (1950). *Tensions affecting international understanding* (Social Science Research Council Bulletin No. 62.). New York: Social Science Research Council.

van Knippenberg, A. (1978). Status differences, comparative relevance and intergroup differentiation. In H. Tajfel (Ed.), *Differentiation between social groups: Studies in the social psychology of intergroup relations.* London: Academic.

van Knippenberg, A., Pruyn, A., & Wilke, H. (1982). Intergroup perceptions in individual and collective encounters. *European Journal of Social Psychology, 12,* 187-193.

van Knippenberg, A. (1984). Intergroup differences in group perceptions. In H. Tajfel (Ed.), *The social dimension: European developments in social psychology* (Vol. 2). Cambridge Paris: Cambridge University Press & Editions de la Maison des Sciences de l'Homme.

Koestler, A. (1969, October 28). Man – one of evolution's mistakes. *New York Times Magazine*, p. 19.

Konečni, V. J. (1979). The role of aversive events in the development of intergroup conflict. In W. Austin & S. Worchel (Eds.), *The social psychology of intergroup relations*. Monterey, CA: Brooks/Cole.

Kravetz, D. F. (1976). Sex role concepts of women. *Journal of Consulting and Clinical Psychology, 44,* 437–443.

Leach, E. R. (1954). *Political systems of highland Burma*. London: Bell.

Le Bon, G. (1897). *The crowd: A study of the popular mind*. London: Unwin.

LeVine, R. A., & Campbell, D. T. (1972). *Ethnocentrism: Theories of conflict, ethnic attitudes and group behavior*. New York: Wiley.

Locksley, A., Hepburn, C., Borgida, E., & Brekke, N. (1980). Sex stereotypes and social judgement. *Journal of Personality and Social Psychology, 39,* 821–831.

Lorenz, K. (1967). *On aggression*. New York: Bantam.

McCauley, C., & Stitt, C. L. (1978). An individual and quantitative measure of stereotypes. *Journal of Personality and Social Psychology, 36,* 929–940.

McDougall, W. (1919). *An introduction to social psychology* (14th ed.). London: Methuen.

Miles, R. (1982). *Racism and migrant labour*. London: Routledge & Kegan Paul.

Milner, D. (1981). Racial prejudice. In J. C. Turner & H. Giles (Eds.), *Intergroup behaviour*. Oxford: Blackwell.

Newcomb, T. M. (1960). Towards an understanding of war. In G. E. Doyle & R. L. Carneiro (Eds.), *Essays in the science of culture*. New York: Crowell.

Ng, S. H. (1982). Power and intergroup discrimination. In H. Tajfel (Ed.), *Social identity and intergroup relations*. Cambridge & Paris: Cambridge University Press and Editions de la Maison des Sciences de l'Homme.

Nye, R. D. (1973). *Conflict among humans: Some basic psychological and social-psychological considerations*. New York: Springer.

Oakes, P. J. (1983). Factors determining the salience of group membership in social perception. Unpublished doctoral thesis, University of Bristol.

Osgood, C. E. (1962). *An alternative to war or surrender*. Urbana, IL: University of Illinois Press.

Parkin, F. (1971). *Class inequality and political order*. London: McGibbon & Kee.

Perkins, T. (1979). Rethinking stereotypes. In M. Barrett, P. Corrigan, A. Kuhn, & J. Wolff (Eds.), *Ideology and cultural production*. London: Croom Helm.

Pettigrew, T. F. (1958). Personality and sociocultural factors in intergroup attitudes: A cross-national comparison. *Journal of Conflict Resolution, 2,* 29.

Pettigrew, T. F. (1981). Extending the stereotype concept. In D. L. Hamilton (Ed.), *Cognitive processes in stereotyping and intergroup behavior*. Hillsdale, NJ: Erlbaum.

Rabbie, J. M., & de Brey, J. H. C. (1971). The anticipation of intergroup cooperation and competition under public and private conditions. *International Journal of Group Tensions, 1,* 230–251.

Rabbie, J. M., & Wilkens, G. (1971). Intergroup competition and its effect on intragroup and intergroup relations. *European Journal of Social Psychology, 1,* 215–234.

Rapoport, A. (1965). Game theory and human conflict. In E. B. McNeil (Ed.), *The nature of human conflict*. Englewood Cliffs, NJ: Prentice-Hall.

Reicher, S. D. (1984, July). *Social identity and social change: Going beyond the elements*. Paper presented at the British Psychological Society (Social Psychology Section) Annual Conference, Oxford.

Reicher, S. D. (1986). Contact, action and racialization: some British evidence. In M. Hewstone & R. J. Brown (Eds.), *Contact and conflict in intergroup encounters*. Oxford: Blackwell.

Roheim, G. (1950). *Psychoanalysis and anthropology: Culture, personality and the unconscious*. New York: International University Press.

Rokeach, M. (1960). *The open and closed mind*. New York: Basic.

Ryen, A. H., & Kahn, A. (1975). Effects of intergroup orientation on group attitudes and proxemic behavior. *Journal of Personality and Social Psychology, 31,* 302–310.

Sanford, N. (1973). Authoritarian personality in contemporary perspective. In J. Knutson (Ed.), *Handbook of political psychology.* San Francisco: Jossey-Bass.

Sherif, M. (1966). *Group conflict and cooperation: Their social psychology.* London: Routledge & Kegan Paul.

Shils, E. (1957). Autoritarianism: 'right' and 'left'. In R. Cristie & M. Jahoda (Eds.), *Studies in the scope and method of the authoritarian personality.* Glencoe, IL: Free Press.

Simmel, G. (1955). *Conflict.* Glencoe, IL: Free Press.

Skevington, S. (1981). Intergroup relations and nursing. *European Journal of Social Psychology, 11,* 43–59.

Snyder, M. (1981). On the self-perpetuating nature of social stereotypes. In D. Hamilton (Ed.), *Cognitive processes in stereotyping and intergroup behavior.* Hillsdale, NJ: Erlbaum.

Stogdill, R. M. (1974). *Handbook of leadership.* New York: Free Press.

Storr, A. (1968). *Human aggression.* Harmondsworth: Penguin.

Sumner, G. A. (1906). *Folkways.* New York: Ginn.

Tajfel, H. (1969). Cognitive aspects of prejudice. *Journal of Social Issues, 25,* 79–97.

Tajfel, H. (1972). Experiments in a vacuum. In J. Israel & H. Tajfel (Eds.), *The context of social psychology: A critical assessment.* London: Academic.

Tajfel, H. (1974). Social identity and intergroup behavior. *Social Science Information, 13,* 65–93.

Tajfel, H. (1977). Social psychology and social reality. *New Society, 39,* 653–654.

Tajfel, H. (Ed.). (1978a). *Differentiation between social groups: Studies in the social psychology of intergroup relations.* London: Academic.

Tajfel, H. (1978b). *The social psychology of minorities.* London: Minority Rights Group.

Tajfel, H. (1979). Human intergroup conflict: Useful and less useful forms of analysis. In M. von Cranach, K. Foppa, W. Lepenies, & D. Ploog (Eds.), *Human ethology: The claims and limits of a new discipline.* Cambridge: Cambridge University Press.

Tajfel, H. (1980). Experimental studies of intergroup behavior. In M. Jeeves (Ed.), *Survey of psychology (No. 3).* London: Allen & Unwin.

Tajfel, H. (1981a). *Human groups and social categories.* Oxford: Blackwell.

Tajfel, H. (1981b). Social stereotypes and social groups. In J. C. Turner & H. Giles (Eds.). *Intergroup behaviour.* Oxford: Basil Blackwell.

Tajfel, H. (1982a). Social psychology of intergroup relations. *Annual Review of Psychology, 33,* 1–39.

Tajfel, H. (Ed.). (1982b). *The social dimension: European developments in social psychology* (Vol. 2). Cambridge and Paris: Cambridge University Press & Editions de la Maison des Sciences de l'Homme.

Tajfel, H., & Turner, J. C. (1979). An integrative theory of intergroup conflict. In W. Austin & S. Worchel (Eds.), *The social psychology of intergroup relations.* Monterey, CA: Brooks/Cole.

Taylor, D., & Simard, L. (1977). *Socially desirable and undesirable consequences of ethnic stereotyping in intergroup relations.* Mimeo, McGill University, Montreal

Taylor, S. E. (1981). A categorization approach to stereotyping. In D. Hamilton (Ed.), *Cognitive processes in stereotyping and intergroup behavior.* Hillsdale, NJ: Erlbaum.

Tropper, R. (1972). The consequences of investment in the process of conflict. *Journal of Conflict Resolution, 16,* 97–98.

Turner, J. C. (1975). Social comparison and social identity: Some prospects for intergroup behaviour. *European Journal of Social Psychology, 5,* 5–34.

Turner, J. C. (1978). Social categorization and social discrimination in the minimal group paradigm. In H. Tajfel (Ed.), *Differentiation between social groups: Studies in the social psychology of intergroup relations.* London: Academic.

Turner, J. C. (1981a). The experimental social psychology of intergroup behaviour. In J. C. Turner & H. Giles (Eds.), *Intergroup behaviour.* Oxford: Blackwell.

Turner, J. C. (1981b). Some considerations in generalizing experimental social psychology. In G. M. Stephenson & J. M. Davis (Eds.), *Progress in applied social psychology* (Vol. 1). London: Wiley.

Turner, J.C. (1982). Towards a cognitive redefinition of the social group. In H. Tajfel (Ed.), *The social dimension: European developments in social psychology* (Vol.2). Cambridge & Paris: Cambridge University Press & Editions de la Maison des Sciences de l'Homme.

Turner, J.C. (1984). Social categorization and the self-concept: A social cognitive theory of group behaviour. In E.J. Lawler (Ed.), *Advances in group processes: Theory and research* (Vol.2). Greenwich, CT: JAI

Turner, J.C., & Brown, R.J. (1978). Social status, cognitive alternatives and intergroup relations. In H. Tajfel (Ed.). *Differentiation between social groups: Studies in the social psychology of intergroup relations.* London: Academic.

Turner, J.C., & Giles, H. (Eds.). (1981). *Intergroup behaviour.* Oxford: Blackwell.

Westergaard, J. (1975). The radical worker. In M. Blumer (Ed.), *Working class images of society.* London & Boston: Routledge & Kegan Paul.

Wetherell, M. (1982). Cross-cultural studies of minimal groups: Implications for the social identity theory of intergroup relations. In H. Tajfel (Ed.), *Social identity and intergroup relations.* Cambridge & Paris: Cambridge University Press & Editions de la Maison des Sciences de l'Homme.

Williams, J. (1984). Gender and intergroup behaviour: Towards an integration. *British Journal of Social Psychology, 23,* 311–316.

Williams, J., & Giles, H. (1978). The changing status of women in society: An intergroup perspective. In H. Tajfel (Ed.), *Differentiation between social groups: Studies in the social psychology of intergroup relations.* London: Academic.

Williams, J., & Morland, J. (1976). *Race, color and the young child.* Chapel Hill: University of North Carolina Press.

Worchel, S., Andreoli, V.A., & Folger, R. (1977). Intergroup cooperation and intergroup attraction: the effect of previous interaction and outcome of combined effort. *Journal of Experimental Social Psychology, 13,* 131–140.

Part II

Cognitive and Motivational Bases of Conflict

Chapter 2

Judgmental Processes as Bases
of Intergroup Conflict

Waldemar Lilli and Jürgen Rehm

Introduction

At first glance, one may wonder whether a social psychological perspective
could be helpful in explaining intergroup and international conflicts, because
there seem to be important differences in their levels of analysis. Conflicts involve groups, institutions, or nations and their relationships, while in social
psychology situations are analyzed primarily on an individual level (Mead,
1934; Stephan, 1985). Theoretically, the aggregation of individual data does not
seem to be sufficient to explain or even to deduce relationships between groups
(see Sherif, 1958; Sherif & Sherif, 1969). Nevertheless, individual judgmental
processes do make important contributions to intergroup and international
conflicts. It is the purpose of this chapter to show this by specifying not only
the extent but also the limitations of these contributions.

Our presentation begins with the most basic and most important cognitive
process in intergroup behavior, namely, the process of categorization. The second section predominantly relies on experimental research in order to lay the
foundations for a deeper understanding of the role of categorization processes
in intergroup conflict. While practical implications will be referred to only occasionally here, they will be of central importance in the subsequent sections.

Additional cognitive processes like deindividuation, illusory correlation,
schema effects, and social comparison are dealt with in the third section, each
of which is followed by at least one example relevant to the intergroup issue.
The reader should be aware that within this section our reasoning always presupposes the basic categorization process.

The fourth section addresses the general impact of cognitive judgmental
processes on conflict phenomena. The contribution of the cognitive perspective
to the prevention and reduction of social conflicts is discussed. The chapter
concludes with speculations about the general role of cognitive judgmental
processes in intergroup and international conflicts.

Categorization

Basic Assumptions

It is evident that in every social conflict at least two distinguishable parties must exist. Participants in a conflict can thus be identified as members of a group, a nation, a tribe, or any other social category.

The first question to be addressed concerns the general psychological consequences of categorization. Classifying objects and people into categories is first of all a powerful means of coping with the overload of information in the environment (see, e.g., Fiske & Taylor, 1984; Taylor, 1981). Categories help us to order the environment and thus enable us to make it meaningful. They also serve as tools for communicating with other persons, allowing the individual to step outside "the silence of the private experience" (Bruner, 1973, p.9). All these advantages, however, seem to be gained at the price of an imperfect image of the world around us (Boulding, 1956), resulting from the necessity of selecting certain aspects of the outside world for information processing.

Second, and more specifically, categorization processes have two consequences: the elements of a single category are usually judged as being more similar than they really are, while elements of different categories are judged as being more dissimilar. Tajfel and Wilkes (1963) called the former an intraclass effect and the latter an interclass effect. Both inter- and intraclass effects have been demonstrated with nonsocial objects (Campbell, 1956; Tajfel & Wilkes, 1963) as well as with social objects. For example, Secord, Bevan, & Katz (1956) found no differences in the degree to which personality traits were attributed to photographs of black persons varying widely in physiognomic negroidness. Having once been categorized as black such a person is seen as having all the typical attributes of this ethnic group even if his or her appearance is Caucasian-like. Moreover, if persons consider this black-white categorization to be very important, they accentuate physiognomic traits as negroid more than members of a control group do. This leads to Conclusion 1.

Conclusion 1: Consequences of general categorization for conflict situations.
Categorization of social and nonsocial objects leads to the perceiving and judging of objects of the same category as more similar to one another than they really are, and enhances perceptual and judgmental contrast between objects of different categories.
Applied to conflicting groups, a disappearance of individual idiosyncracies and differences is to be predicted. Increased anonymity and undifferentiated treatment of individuals will occur.

To demonstrate the applicability of the categorization process, relevant experimental work will be presented in the next section.

Experimental Work Relevant to Basic Categorization Processes

Tajfel and associates (Tajfel, 1959a, 1959b; Tajfel & Wilkes, 1963) developed a basic theory and an experimental paradigm for research in this area. Their main thesis was that inter- and intraclass effects occur regularly if a continuous stimulus dimension is superimposed by a classification scheme (the term "classification" here indicates a subcase of categorization, that is, the respective categories break one or more continuous stimulus dimension(s) into parts).

In his book on stereotyping, Lilli (1982) investigated the implications of this concept for the ananlysis of social categorization processes in a series of experiments. He dealt with additional restrictive conditions for the classification process (e. g., anchoring of the judgmental scale, cognitive complexity) and its application in more realistic settings (e.g., in the perception of faces or in judgments of political parties and candidates during an election campaign). The major thrust of Lilli's work, however, was the consideration of three principal questions which will be discussed below:

1. Is it a necessary condition for the occurrence of classification effects that the stimulus-classification correspondence is perfect? What degree of regularity is sufficient for classification?
2. Will the inter- and intraclass effects also occur with social stimuli and emotionally relevant classifications? Are these similarity and contrast effects observable in complex settings?
3. If the relationship between stimulus dimension and classification is the result of learning processes, what implications does this have for the stability of resulting judgments? Is a classification (e. g., Russians are aggressive/Americans are peaceful), once learned, irreversible?

The first issue was addressed in a series of experiments on the variation of the stimulus dimension-classification covariation. Before Lilli's work, experiments on classification nearly always studied perfect relationships between a stimulus dimension and classification. The original study by Tajfel and Wilkes (1963), for example, used eight different lengths of lines as stimuli, where the four shorter lines carried the letter A, the longer, the letter B. This led us to the question as to what would happen under conditions of less than perfect relationships? To test this empirically, five different stimulus-classification relationships were created, ranging from perfect to random cases.

Numerically, these relationships can be described by their respective probabilities, ranging from 1.0 (perfect correspondence) to 0.5 (random) with steps at 0.92 (nearly perfect), 0.83 (moderate correspondence), and 0.68 (nearly random). As in the study of Tajfel and Wilkes (1963), the stimuli consisted of eight different lengths of lines, and the classification used the letters A and B. Within this design the letters corresponded more or less strongly to the four longer lines; the classification should thus have been more or less useful in estimating the length of the lines. All five levels of this independent factor were presented to different groups of subjects in a training phase, when subjects learned the stimulus-classification relationship assigned to them. In the subsequent test phase, subjects had to judge the length of the randomly presented lines in centimeters. The results showed that substantial interclass effects occur only under the $p = 1.0$ and the $p = 0.92$ conditions, indicating that, as postulated, a nearly perfect relationship between stimuli and classification is necessary to produce inter- and intraclass effects.

The second issue was addressed in a set of experiments on the complexity of stimuli and emotionality of classification. The aim of these experiments was to show that inter- and intraclass effects also occur if more complex stimuli are to be judged. This would demonstrate the applicability of the classification theory to categorization of social objects as well.

Two different series of faces, varying in height of the forehead, were used as stimuli. One series consisted of schematic, the other of more realistic, and thus more complex, faces (photograph quality). Two classification conditions were introduced: first, the well-known A-B classification, and, second, a more realistic classification represented by the notions of "blue" versus "white-collar" workers. In a training phase, perfect correlations ($p = 1.0$) between the labels A (blue-collar worker) and the lower foreheads and between B (white-collar worker) and the higher foreheads were established. In one of these experiments, subjects had to estimate the "intelligence" of the presented faces.

Results showed at least a tendency for classification effects to be greater if more complex stimulus situations were given. They also seem to generalize to subjectively related attributes like perceived intelligence. Since conflict situations are of high complexity, stronger classification effects can be expected here. Furthermore, a study by Marchand (1970) clearly showed that emotionally relevant classifications produced substantially greater effects than neutral ones. While conflict situations are assumed to be characterized by emotionalization, straightforward classifications may govern the respective cognitive processes.

To answer the third question, a number of experiments on the stability of classification judgments were conducted. The main issue addressed in these experiments was whether a stimulus-classification relationship, once learned, would be so rigid that under the extreme condition of an inversion of the relationship, subjects would not relearn the new classification.

A series of faces were again used as stimuli, this time constructed on the basis of a police card index for the identification of criminals. A series with six different faces was obtained by varying the height of the forehead; again, the letters A and B formed the classification. Seven groups of subjects were tested according to different stimulus dimension-classification relationships, again made operational in terms of different covariation conditions. Groups were exposed to various conditions ($p = 1.0$; 0.96; 0.83; 0.75; 0.67, or 0.5) in a training phase, while a control group had no training. Subjects were asked to estimate the height of the foreheads.

Only the first 24 presentations of the test phase were in accordance with the covariation conditions presented in the training phase. Subjects were not informed about subsequent changes in covariation conditions ($p = -1.0$). For the subjects in the $p = 1.0$ group this was a complete reversal of learned relationships. Subjects in other groups were confronted with increasing levels of contradiction along the increasing stimulus-classification probabilities learned during the training phase.

Results clearly showed that the subjects maintained the once learned relationship, and went on trying to apply it to the new situation; even under the weak covariation conditions, a relearning was not observed. These results strongly support the hypothesis that, once-learned, a categorical division of stimuli cannot easily be abandoned and replaced by another solution, even if more adequate.

These findings may shed some light on existing classifications held by conflicting parties or nations concerning their respective enemies. For example, if this notion is applicable to the conflict between Iran and Iraq, there would be little hope of ending the war by trying to alter the mutually held classification.

Conclusion 2: Limiting conditions to the categorization process.
Interclass and intraclass effects of categorization occur only under a nearly perfect and visible covariation between stimuli and superimposed categories. They are strengthened by more complex stimulus situations and maintained even if a previously learned covariation is not really applicable to stimulus situations.

Consequences of Social Categorization

So far the discussion has focused on the basic categorization processes showing an individual judging social objects. Do the principles of this process apply to all situations? To answer this question, our discussion will now focus on the *social context* of the individual judge, especially the judge's relevant group memberships. The main question at this point concerns the determination of judgments as a result of affiliation due to membership in certain groups. The term "social categorization" is now used in its full meaning as the judgment of social objects in social contexts. While in the previous perspective the judgmental effects consisted of similarities and dissimilarities between objects, evaluative aspects are now of primary interest.

Many experiments, and everyday observations as well, show that social categorizations are often followed by positive ingroup and negative outgroup evaluations (see Brewer, 1979, for an overview), which achieve stability especially in cases where no opportunities exist to change group membership (Tajfel, 1981). The so-called minimal group research initiated by Tajfel, Billig, Bundy, and Flament (1971) measured some of the behavioral effects of being divided into groups. This paradigm has the following characteristics: (a) a division of subjects into categories (groups) according to irrelevant criteria (e.g., preferences for pictures, estimations of dots); (b) no face-to-face interactions within and between groups; (c) anonymity of group membership; (d) rewards and punishments distributed on the group level only.

Results of minimal group studies consistently showed that subjects typically chose a strategy of ingroup favoritism. For example, subjects tried to maximize the reward *differences* between their ingroup and the outgroup, even if strategies like "fairness" (equal rewards for ingroup and outgroup), "maximum joint profit" for both groups, or "maximum payoff" for the ingroup were also available (Tajfel et al., 1971; Billig & Tajfel, 1973). Furthermore, it was found that groups formed by random assignment of subjects led to considerably more marked discrimination compared with groups formed by a division of subjects in terms of interindividual similarities.

Similar ingroup favoritism was obtained in many other studies with different operationalizations for the independent as well as for the dependent variables (Brewer, 1979). Most importantly, ingroup biases have also been replicated for evaluative trait ratings of groups. It should further be noted that "any of the situational factors found to be associated with enhancement of in-group bias can be subsumed under the effect of the salience of the distinction between in-group and out-group" (Brewer, 1979, p.319).

The main point here concerns the fact that *cognitive factors can apparently influence or even cause subsequent evaluations*. However, such evaluations do not always favor the ingroup. Under certain conditions, individuals have to accept negative evaluations of their own group (e.g., self-hatred among Jews: Lewin, 1953; or "soiled identity" among blacks in the USA during the 1940s and 1950s: Pettigrew, 1983, p.52). These arguments are summarized in Conclusion 3.

Conclusion 3: Evaluative consequences of social categorization for intergroup conflict.
Social categorization leads to evaluative judgments about in- and outgroup(s). This effect occurs even if individuals are categorized according to irrelevant criteria. At times of conflict, categorization effects become even more prominent and produce strong positive ingroup biases.

The last sentence of Conclusion 3 needs some further elaboration. First of all, it should be noted that there are significant structural analogies between minimal group situations and conflict situations; they have in common that the individuals involved are confronted with a radical dichotomy existing between their own membership and another category. This phenomenon is called *simple categorization* by Deschamps and Doise (1978). If somebody belongs to one party, he cannot at the same time belong to the other party in that conflict. Furthermore, in both cases there is no opportunity to change group membership. In sum, salience of categories, division into mutually exclusive groups, and limitations of free membership choice all together result in an enhancement of the positiveness of the ingroup.

A further important and more general consequence of social categorization is that it provides individuals with a system of orientations towards their social world. Social categories "create and define the individual's place in society" (Tajfel & Turner, 1979, p.40; see also Tajfel, 1981) and provide them with an identification in social terms. Under certain circumstances, however, individuals find their search for a positive social identity thwarted. For instance, their own category, their ingroup, may be the object of a new (negative) interpretation (e.g., living in Harlem is often identified with being criminal). An even more extreme case arises when individuals are personally labeled or put into negatively evaluated categories to which the individuals themselves do not feel that they belong. Depending on the degree of threat a stigmatization has for social identity, conflicts may be initiated by the affected people. Recent uprisings in the Republic of South Africa give an example of a negatively labeled (majority) group, trying to make a stand (Prus, 1975). Of course, other factors also contributed to these uprisings (see the next section for a more detailed discussion).

Conclusion 4: Resistance to negative categorization.
Resistance to being negatively categorized (labeled) may cause conflicts.

So far, the foundations of *categorization processes* relevant to conflict have been outlined. While categorization is the most basic and necessary condition for the development and maintenance of conflicts, some additional processes are needed to complete the social psychological analysis of this issue. Therefore, a discussion of supplementary cognitive phenomena follows in the next section.

Supplementary Cognitive Processes and Their Contribution to the Study of Intergroup and International Conflict

Four additional cognitive phenomena relevant to the social psychological analysis of conflict will be discussed in this section. These are: *deindividuation,* which may cause aggressive acts against the outgroup; *illusory correlation* and *schema effects,* which may contribute to the formation and/or maintenance of negative outgroup images; and *social comparison* processes, which may contribute to the justification of conflicts in several ways.

Since these phenomena and processes are of a basic cognitive nature, at least two limitations should be kept in mind. Firstly, conflicts are initiated and maintained by noncognitive (e.g., economic) conditions as well. Secondly, our knowledge about the effects of cognitive processes stems mainly from experimental research and should therefore be applied with due caution. Moreover, theoretically necessary antecedent conditions are seldom found in pure form in social realities (Gadenne, 1984; Manicas & Secord, 1983). Nevertheless, the insight gained from the study of social cognition is important for our understanding of the dynamics of social conflicts, especially with respect to their initiation, maintenance, and justification (see also Hewstone, this volume).

Deindividuation

As we have seen, categorization leads to accentuation of similarity between members of the same group (intraclass effect). Thus, individual idiosyncracies and differences within a group disappear to some degree, strengthening the perception of anonymity (see Conclusion 1 above). This development results in a kind of deindividuation, which Festinger, Pepitone & Newcomb (1952, p. 389) described as a phenomenon in which group members do not pay attention to other members as individuals and also do not feel that they are singled out as individuals by others. Deindividuation was found to reduce inner restraints of group members (Festinger et al., 1952), which sometimes results in aggressive acts (Zimbardo, 1969).

Steinleitner (1985) tested this deindividuation-aggression hypothesis in situations of intergroup competition, using games of volleyball. To experimentally induce intraclass similarity he distributed T-shirts of a striking yellow color to the members of one of the two competing teams. Members of the other team wore their own individual shirts which differed widely in color and style. As predicted, the teams with greater visible intraclass similarity (more deindividuated groups) showed significantly more aggressive acts (fouls) than the non deindividuated teams in the 30 games that were observed.

Another study showed that this deindividuation-aggression relationship can also be widely found in natural settings: Watson (1973) correlated reports about deindividuation mechanisms within tribes of different cultures (body and face marking, special garments or hairstyles) with reports about aggressive acts of these tribes and obtained significant results.

Such deindividuation mechanisms are prevalent in times of war, where members of the same party wear the same uniforms. Uniforms as well as other measures to increase intraclass effects can thus be understood as applied cases of categorization theory. Of course, such measures were most often employed for other reasons, without consideration of their cognitive and behavioral consequences.

Conclusion 5: Categorization and deindividuation.
Strong intraclass effects result in deindividuation, which facilitates the conduct of aggressive acts toward outgroups. Under certain conditions, deindividuation mechanisms can initiate conflicts; they always seem to escalate them.

Illusory Correlation

The term "illusory correlation" refers to a cognitive process in which two classes of events are perceived as belonging together, which in reality (a) are not correlated at all, or (b) are correlated to a much weaker degree than perceived (Chapman, 1967). In her original paper about illusory correlations in verbal learning tasks, Chapman (1967) states two possible conditions for their occurrence: (1) associativeness and (2) distinctiveness.

In studies relevant to conflict research, *associativeness* has mostly been put into operation by using stereotypes, for example, culturally formed associations between group membership and some negative attributes (see, e.g., Hamilton & Rose, 1980; McArthur & Friedman, 1980). The *distinctiveness* factor is conveniently operationalized as the relative infrequency of events within the context of a stimulus set (Hamilton, Dugan, & Trolier, 1985; Hamilton & Gifford, 1976; Spears, van der Pligt, & Eiser, 1985; Tversky & Kahneman, 1974).

What are the implications of this research for the study of intergroup relations? Consider the case where a minority group is negatively stereotyped by majority group members. Such stereotypical statements can, in most cases, be interpreted as a correlation between group membership and some negative attribute or negative behaviors (see Hamilton, 1981, p. 116f.): blacks are lazy, Turks are dirty and criminal, Germans are militaristic. For statements like this, the concept of illusory correlation would predict:

1. An *already existing negative stereotype* (e.g., in Germany: Russians are aggressive) will be maintained or strengthened due to its (cognitive) *associative bonds* between group membership and negative attributes (behaviors), even if the individual judge does not encounter information confirming such a relationship (see, e.g., Hamilton & Rose, 1980).
2. An *existing negative stereotype about a minority group* (e.g., Turks are criminal) will be strengthened by *distinctiveness* of the two relevant events: first, the minority group in most cases can be considered as distinctive because interactions with members of that group are statistically relatively infrequent occurrences (additionally, minority group members are often visibly distinctive, e.g., by the color of their skin or by other physical attributes; see, e.g., Hawley, 1944, or LeVine & Campbell, 1972). Second, negatively judged behaviors, such as criminal acts, quite often violate social norms and usually occur more infrequently compared to positively judged, desirable behaviors, thus becoming more distinctive. The concept of illusory correlation would predict that the coincidence of these two distinctive factors will be overestimated, leading to the strengthening of negative stereotypes above described (see, e.g., McArthur & Friedman, 1980).
3. Even if a negative stereotype does not already exist, it may be formed due to the coincidence of the *distinctive factors* (see, e.g., Hamilton & Gifford, 1976; Hamilton et al., 1985).

Some limiting conditions of illusory correlation processes should not be overlooked here. First, illusory correlation biases take place only during the encoding of serially presented information, that is, if combinations of group/attribute information are displayed successively (cf. Hamilton et al., 1985). But this is a condition quite often characteristic of intergroup situations, where members of one group acquire information from time to time about behaviors of outgroup members. Second, complexity and transparency of the judgmental situation both play an important role. In situations of less transparency, illusory correlation biases are strengthened (Lilli & Rehm, 1984). Usually, judgments about social groups are by no means simple, nor are they based on information from good authority. Third, preexisting, conflicting stereotypes in the opposite direction can prevent the formation of stereotypic beliefs due to distinctiveness-based illusory correlation effects (McArthur & Friedman, 1980). Almost all of these boundary conditions, however, seem to be fulfilled in judgments about outgroup members. Therefore, in such situations, we would expect illusory correlation biases to occur, often resulting in the persistence of negative stereotypes about the outgroup.

So far, we have dealt only with stereotypes without explicitly mentioning their relationship to conflict. In this respect, two points deserve further consideration:

1. Negative stereotypes about the enemies in a conflict are of *functional* value, because they offer justifications for maintaining conflicts (see Tajfel, 1981; for economic conflicts, Levin, 1975).
2. Negative stereotypes about an outgroup can help to start a conflict. This may be the case if members of one group start acting in line with their judgments. This brings us back to the old attitude-behavior issue: under what conditions does prejudice lead to discriminatory behavior and/or social conflict? In an attempt to address this issue Grimshaw (1969, p.452) suggested some limiting conditions. He argued that negative attitudes about outgroups would only lead to social violence and conflict if there were social tension and weak external controls. Though Grimshaw's idea is not unproblematic (Rehm, 1986), it could be a useful basis for more systematic research in this area.

Conclusion 6: Consequences of illusory correlation for intergroup conflicts.
The phenomenon of illusory correlation can contribute to an explanation of the formation and persistence of social stereotypes, thus improving our understanding of conflict initiation and maintenance.

One historical example may demonstrate possible contributions of illusory correlations to conflict issues: in 1947, when the states of India and Pakistan were founded, thousands of Muslims crossed over the new border towards Pakistan, while thousands of Hindus were heading in the opposite direction. During these movements social tensions arose, sometimes resulting in mutual aggressive acts (e.g., throwing of stones). In situations like this an overestimation of aggressive acts by the outgroup can be predicted, enhancing mutual negative stereotypes.

Schema Effects

Most cognitive processes, including categorization, should be conceived as useful tools for coping with the complexity of our informational environment. When, however, in certain cases, they become overgeneralized, errors and biases occur (Nisbett & Ross, 1980). From this perspective, one cannot speak of "correct" or "incorrect" outcomes of cognitive processes, but only of their adequate or inadequate application. Consider, for example, the encoding of information about in- and outgroups. Since we usually expect there to be more contacts with ingroup members, it really seems to be functional and adequate to memorize more detailed and differentiated information about these people. It can be assumed that this is achieved by different encoding strategies: while information about ingroups is encoded on a subcategorical, differentiated and individual level, superordinate, undifferentiated, and general categories are used to encode information about outgroups (Park & Rothbart, 1982; Rehm, 1984).

The disadvantages of this memorizing process are twofold. First of all, it results in a more homogeneous and less informative schema or image of the outgroup (Park & Rothbart, 1982). Conflict can thus be justified and maintained by pitting the more complex ingroup schema against an undifferentiated outgroup schema. Second, as Linville (1982; see also Linville & Jones, 1980) has shown, less complex schemata lead to more polarized *evaluations*. Given the case that moderately negative behavior is displayed by a member of the outgroup, quite extreme negative judgments will follow (compared to judgments about the same behavior shown by an ingroup member).

Conclusion 7: Social categorization and complexity of ingroup vs. outgroup schemata.
Social categorization leads to different encoding strategies for information about in- and outgroups, resulting in different schemata. These differences of schemata can be seen as background for arguments to maintain and justify conflicts.

Social Comparison Processes

Although social comparison processes are usually not seen exclusively from a cognitive perspective, our argument for referring to them here comes from the consideration that comparisons often seem to designate the next steps following social categorizations within the sequence of processes leading to conflicts. In other words, individual perceptions of belonging to a social category are necessary prerequisites for subsequent social comparisons.

While the original version of social comparison theory (Festinger, 1950, 1954) analyzed individual comparisons *within* groups (an aspect not covered here), the social identity theory developed by Tajfel (1981, p.254f.) focused on comparison *between* groups, which is an aspect of major importance in the present discussion. Most characteristics of one's group as a whole can be assessed only in relation to perceived differences from other groups and their implied value connotations. If we assume that individuals try to uphold positive social identities (Tajfel & Turner, 1979), the result is a devaluation of the outgroup in situations of conflict. Sometimes the only way of achieving this goal is by comparison with others less fortunate (downward comparison principle, Wills, 1981), especially in cases where social identity is attacked.

In what way do social comparisons conceivably contribute to the initiation of conflicts? From the perspective of the social identity principle (Tajfel & Turner, 1979) and the downward comparison principle (Wills, 1981), any attempt by members of a lower status group to improve their social identities should lead to the following consequences:

First, group members may find an even less fortunate group to compare with and thus restore subjective well-being. Unfortunately, this results in a further devaluation of the comparison target group. The recent increase of prejudicial judgments against Turkish immigrant workers by unemployed Germans in the Federal Republic is an example. The devaluation of the target may even escalate to aggressive acts, e.g., recent arson attacks against Turkish dwellings in Germany.

Subjective well-being may possibly be restored directly by doing harm to others (Wills, 1981). Currently, the targets of these aggressive acts are not at all adequately predicted by social psychological theories. If a member of a group is attacked by an outgroup member, the group as a whole might feel threatened, and therefore ingroup solidarity and awareness of group identity may be strengthened (Coser, 1956; Sherif, Harvey, White, Hood, & Sherif, 1961). On the other hand, members of the group to which the aggressor belongs may declare themselves supportive of this action. The end of such a vicious circle will be mutual devaluation and its escalation may lead to a conflict between the engaged groups. An experimental example is given by Donnerstein, Donnerstein, Simon, & Ditrichs (1972); they found an increasing number of aggressive acts toward blacks following a campus racial disturbance. A tragic example of cyclical aggression in intergroup conflict is illustrated by the events following the murder of the Indian prime minister, Indira Gandhi.

So far, we have only considered cases in which intergroup conflicts are possible outcomes while mutual devaluations are certain. A third alternative should not be overlooked. This concerns reassessments of ingroup traits. A very famous example for this was the 'black is beautiful' movement, an enterprise which successfully established a strong and proud minority (Pettigrew, 1983; see also Tajfel, 1981). This is a case where comparisons mainly take place within, and less frequently between, groups. But the result of self-enhancements can finally end in a revival of aggressive acts under a changed name. This line of reasoning is summarized in Conclusion 8.

Conclusion 8: Initiations of intergroup conflict by social comparison processes.
If social identity is improved by downward comparisons, under some circumstances mutual devaluations and intergroup conflicts can result.

Obviously the value of this assumption is rather restricted; further limiting conditions are indeed necessary to specify improved versions of social identity theory. But we are not very optimistic that intergroup problems of this kind can be adequately addressed under the "sovereignty of social cognition" alone, to use the phraseology of Ostrom (1984).

To be sure, comparison processes serve to maintain and justify social conflicts as well. The theory of informal social communication (Festinger, 1950; Irle, 1985) concentrates on corresponding processes within groups. According to Festinger, pressures upon members toward uniformity will be exercised if there is a functional necessity for goal attainment. At times of conflict, unanimity in negative evaluations and actions against the outgroup is not only extremely functional but also often a prerequisite for winning the conflict. Parts of this communication process (directed, for instance, toward doubtful ingroup members) consist of extremely rigid negative outgroup images. The more these informal procedures are carried out by organized actions, the greater will be their success.

Conclusion 9: Justification and maintenance of conflicts through social comparison processes.
Efforts toward uniformity and increasing social control within the groups engaged are sources of the maintenance and justification of the conflict situation.

General Impact of Cognitive Judgmental Processes on Conflict Phenomena

So far, we have discussed different cognitive processes and their implications and consequences for situations of conflict. In this section an attempt will be made to evaluate their joint contribution to the analysis of conflict.

It is a truism to say that cognitive processes are processes which take place within individuals. But it is no less true that the agents in conflict situations are typically individuals who have great influence with the public. Politicians and political actors have the power to communicate conflict-related categorizations so that a consensus among people is likely to occur. Hitler in Germany and Khomeini in Iran are prominent examples of this. There is no doubt that the enforced communication of suitable ingroup/outgroup schemata by Hitler and Khomeini can be understood as one of the most important prerequisites of the subsequent conflicts. Ingroup/outgroup schemata of that kind (or comparable categorizations), once extended, apparently need constant reinforcement in order to perpetuate their salience as justifications for holding an existing conflict alive. In this respect, we are sure that both the development of special categorizations or schemata *and* their communication to the people involved are an important part of the rules of the game of staging conflicts. This is true at the levels of groups and nations as well. The groups participating in an overt (or even a covert) conflict can be characterized by communication that remains predominantly, if not even totally, within their own belief systems. The result is that little or no information about the outgroup enters the exclusive circle of communication. This vacuum tends to be filled by self-produced information about the outgroup which serves to confirm the position of the ingroup. As the categorization experiments have shown, the mutually held categories need not be realistic; the essential issue concerns the perception/cognition of a strong relationship between stimulus (e.g., outgroup) and classification (e.g., to be aggressive).

There are some examples in the history of mankind which show the persistence of conflict-related categories long after the conflict itself has ended. After the Second World War, this was definitely the case in the relationship between

Germany and France. Though historical explanations may be plausible, it is a *psychological* fact that well-learned categories are not easily extinguished. There are, however, some ways to weaken conflict-related categories. The two most important ones seem to be (a) the crossing of categorizations and (b) the re-opening of the exclusive communication circles and mutual information exchange under conditions of an external or internal pressure towards a change of the situation.

After the Second World War, in both Germany and France, the old conflict-supporting images still existed. Recent survey data, however, show convincingly that the French and Germans nowadays regard one another in a much more differentiated and positive way. Findings reported by Deschamps and Doise (1978) on the impact of crossed category memberships in intergroup relations suggest that this development could be due to the fact that the importance of the old categorization is crossed by other categories. As many exchange programs between these countries were established, pupils of the same age and educational level, for example, came together, as well as sports clubs and other associations from both nations. As a result, these new categories become more prominent to the participants in the programs and the effect of the old categories is reduced (but see also Stroebe, Lenkert, & Jonas, this volume). This example points to the importance of the availability of meaningful new categories which overlap the old ones.

The assumption that the mutually held categorizations of the parties in conflict are partly the result of exclusive communication circles points to the necessity of these circles' being reopened to set basic situational changes into action. Since Sherif's field experiments with young boys in vacation camps, we are aware of the possibility of bringing both parties together, if a task can be found which is of comparably high importance for both and can only be solved by cooperation of both sides (but see Condor & Brown, this volume).

Is it not conceivable that the solution of urgent ecological problems could be perceived as a task of mutual importance by both East and West? A second possibility could be the interference of a third, mediating party; but as some dramatic examples of our times show, this model too often leads to an escalation of conflict rather than to its reduction.

Cognitive processes like those we have dealt with in this paper play a supporting, rather than a reducing, role in different stages of conflict. This is mainly due to their inherent characteristics: categorizations and additional cognitive processes are results of highly selective information processes. Systematic errors and biases may thus rule the situation. Empirical evidence and observations of real existing conflicts in our world support this notion.

References

Billig, M., & Tajfel, H. (1973). Social categorization and similarity in intergroup behavior. *European Journal of Social Psychology, 3*, 27–52.

Boulding, K. E. (1956). *The Image*. Ann Arbor: University of Michigan Press.

Brewer, M. B. (1979). In-group bias in the minimal intergroup situation: A cognitive-motivational analysis. *Psychological Bulletin, 86*, 307–324.

Bruner, J. S. (1973). *Going beyond the information given*. New York: Norton.

Campbell, D. T. (1956). Enhancement of contrast as composite habit. *Journal of Abnormal and Social Psychology, 53*, 350–355.

Chapman, L. J. (1967). Illusory correlation in observational report. *Journal of Verbal Learning and Verbal Behavior, 6*, 151–153.

Coser, L. A. (1956). *The Functions of social conflict*. Glencoe, IL: Free Press.

Deschamps, J.-C., & Doise, W. (1978). Crossed category memberships in intergroup relations. In H. Tajfel (Ed.), *Differentiations between social groups: Studies in the social psychology of intergroup relations* (pp. 141–158). London: Academic.

Donnerstein, E., Donnerstein, M., Simon, S., & Ditrichs, R. (1972). Variables in interracial aggression: Anonymity, expected retaliation, and a riot. *Journal of Personality and Social Psychology, 22*, 236–245.

Festinger, L. (1950). Informal social communication. *Psychological Review, 57*, 271–282.

Festinger, L. (1954). A theory of social comparison processes. *Human Relations, 7*, 117–140.

Festinger, L., Pepitone, A., & Newcomb, T. (1952). Some consequences of deindividuation in a group. *Journal of Abnormal and Social Psychology, 47*, 382–389.

Fiske, S. T., & Taylor, S. E. (1984). *Social cognition*. Reading, MA: Addison-Wesley.

Gadenne, V. (1984). *Theorie und Erfahrung in der psychologischen Forschung*. Tübingen: Mohr.

Grimshaw, A. D. (1969). Relationship among prejudice, discrimination, social tension, and social violence. In A. D. Grimshaw (Ed.), *Racial violence in the United States* (pp. 446–454). Chicago: Aldine.

Hamilton, D. L. (1981). Illusory correlation as a basis for stereotyping. In D. L. Hamilton (Ed.), *Cognitive processes in stereotyping and intergroup behavior* (pp. 115–144). Hillsdale, NJ: Erlbaum.

Hamilton, D. L., Dugan, P. M., & Trolier, T. K. (1985). The formation of stereotypic beliefs: Further evidence for distinctiveness-based illusory correlations. *Journal of Personality and Social Psychology, 48*, 5–17.

Hamilton, D. L., & Gifford, R. K. (1976). Illusory correlation in interpersonal perception: A cognitive basis of stereotypic judgments. *Journal of Experimental Social Psychology, 12*, 392–407.

Hamilton, D. L., & Rose, T. L. (1980). Illusory correlation and the maintenance of stereotypic beliefs. *Journal of Personality and Social Psychology, 39*, 832–845.

Hawley, A. H. (1944). Dispersion versus segregation. Apropos a solution of race problems. *Papers of the Michigan Academy of Science, Arts, and Letters, 30*, 667–674.

Irle, M. (1985). Konvergenz und Divergenz in Gruppen. In D. Frey & M. Irle (Eds.), *Theorien der Sozialpsychologie, Band II: Gruppen- und Lerntheorien*. Bern: Huber.

Levin, J. (1975). *The function of prejudice*. New York: Harper & Row.

LeVine, R. A., & Campbell, D. T. (1972). *Ethnocentrism: Theories of conflict, ethnic attitudes, and group behavior*. New York: Wiley.

Lewin, K. (1953). Psychosoziologische Probleme einer Minderheitengruppe. In G. W. Lewin (Ed.), *Die Lösung sozialer Konflikte. Ausgewählte Abhandlungen über Gruppendynamik* (pp. 204–221). Bad Nauheim, FRG: Christian.

Lilli, W. (1982). *Grundlagen der Stereotypisierung*. Göttingen: Hogrefe.

Lilli, W., & Rehm, J. (1984). Theoretische und empirische Untersuchungen zum Phänomen der Zusammenhangstäuschung. II. Entwicklung eines Modells zum quantitativen Urteil und Diskussion seiner Implikationen für die soziale Urteilsbildung. *Zeitschrift für Sozialpsychologie, 15*, 60–73.

Linville, P. W. (1982). The complexity-extremity effect and age-based stereotyping. *Journal of Personality and Social Psychology, 42,* 193–211.

Linville, P. W., & Jones, E. E. (1980). Polarized appraisals of out-group members. *Journal of Personality and Social Psychology, 38,* 689–703.

Manicas, P. T., & Secord, P. F. (1983). Implications for psychology of the new philosophy of science. *American Psychologist, 38,* 399–413.

Marchand, B. (1970). Auswirkung einer emotional wertvollen und einer emotional neutralen Klassifikation auf die Schätzung einer Stimulusserie. *Zeitschrift für Sozialpsychologie, 1,* 264–274.

McArthur, L. Z., & Friedman, S. A. (1980). Illusory correlation in impression formation: Variations in the shared distinctiveness effect as a function of the distinctive person's age, race, and sex. *Journal of Personality and Social Psychology, 39,* 615–624.

Mead, G. H. (1934). *Mind, self, and society.* Chicago: University of Chicago Press.

Nisbett, R. R., & Ross, L. (1980). *Human inference: Strategies and shortcomings of social judgement.* Englewood Cliffs, NJ: Prentice-Hall.

Ostrom, T. M. (1984). The sovereignty of social cognition. In R. S. Wyer & T. K. Srull (Eds.), *Handbook of social cognition* (Vol. 1, pp. 1–38). Hillsdale, NJ: Erlbaum.

Park, B., & Rothbart, M. (1982). Perception of out-group homogeneity and levels of social categorization: Memory for the subordinate attributes of in-group and out-group members. *Journal of Personality and Social Psychology, 42,* 1051–1068.

Pettigrew, T. F. (1983). Group identity and social comparisons. In C. Fried (Ed.), *Minorities: Community and identity* (pp. 51–60). Berlin: Springer.

Prus, R. C. (1975). Labeling-theory: A reconceptualization and a propositional statement on typing. *Sociological Focus, 8,* 79–96.

Rehm, J. (1984). *Kognitive Prozesse bei der Vorurteilsbildung.* Unpublished Diplomarbeit, Mannheim University.

Rehm, J. (1986). Theoretische und methodologische Probleme bei der Erforschung von Vorurteilen, I and II. *Zeitschrift für Sozialpsychologie, 17,* 18–30, 74–86.

Rothbart, M., Dawes, R., & Park, B. (1984). Stereotyping and sampling biases in intergroup perception. In J. R. Eiser (Ed.), *Attitudinal Judgment* (pp. 109–134). New York: Springer.

Secord, P. F., Bevan, W., & Katz, B. (1956). The negro stereotype and perceptual accentuation. *Journal of Abnormal and Social Psychology, 53,* 78–83.

Sherif, M. (1958). Superordinate goals in the reduction of intergroup conflicts. *American Journal of Sociology, 63,* 349–356.

Sherif, M., Harvey, O. J., White, B. J., Hood, W. R., & Sherif, C. W. (1961). *Intergroup conflict and cooperation: The robbers' cave experiment.* Norman: University of Oklahoma Press.

Sherif, M., & Sherif, C. W. (1969). *Social psychology.* New York: Harper.

Spears, R., van der Pligt, J., & Eiser, J. R. (1985). Illusory correlation in the perception of group attitudes. *Journal of Personality and Social Psychology, 48,* 863–875.

Steinleitner, M. (1985). *Aggression and Deindividuation in Gruppen (-situationen). Eine experimentelle Studie.* Unpublished Diplomarbeit, Mannheim University.

Stephan, W. G. (1985). Intergroup relations. In G. Lindzey & E. Aronson (Eds.), *The handbook of social psychology* (pp. 599–658). New York: Random House.

Tajfel, H. (1959a). Quantitative judgment in social perception. *British Journal of Psychology, 50,* 16–29.

Tajfel, H. (1959b). The anchoring effects of value in a scale of judgements. *British Journal of Psychology, 50,* 294–304.

Tajfel, H. (1974). Social identity and intergroup behavior. *Social Science Information, 13,* 65–93.

Tajfel, H. (1981). *Human groups and social categories: Studies in social psychology.* Cambridge: Cambridge University Press.

Tajfel, H., Billig, M. G., Bundy, R. P., & Flament, C. (1971). Social categorization and intergroup behavior. *European Journal of Social Psychology, 1,* 149–178.

Tajfel, H., & Turner, J. (1979). An integrative theory of intergroup conflict. In W. G. Austin & S. Worchel (Eds.), *The social psychology of intergroup relations* (pp. 33–47). Monterey, CA: Brooks/Cole.

Tajfel, H., & Wilkes, A. L. (1963). Classification and quantitative judgement. *British Journal of Psychology, 54,* 101–114.

Taylor, S. E. (1981). A categorization approach to stereotyping. In D. L. Hamilton (Ed.), *Cognitive processes in stereotyping and intergroup behavior* (pp. 83–114). Hillsdale, NJ: Erlbaum.

Tversky, A., & Kahneman, D. (1974). Judgment under uncertainty: Heuristics and biases. *Science, 185,* 1124–1131.

Watson, R. I. (1973). Investigation into Deindividuation using a cross-cultural survey technique. *Journal of Personality and Social Psychology, 25,* 342–345.

Wills, T. A. (1981). Downward comparison principles in social psychology. *Psychological Bulletin, 90,* 245–271.

Zimbardo, P. G. (1969). The human choice: Individuation, reason, and order versus deindividuation, impulse, and chaos. In W. J. Arnold & D. LeVine (Eds.), *Nebraska Symposium on Motivation* (pp. 237–307). Lincoln: University of Nebraska Press.

Chapter 3

Attributional Bases of Intergroup Conflict

Miles Hewstone

> As long as groups are in conflict, the casting of blame by either side will lead to a vicious circle of mutual recriminations.
> Muzafer Sherif, 1966, p.115

Introduction

Although many definitions of intergroup conflict include an emphasis on incompatible goals and limited resources (e.g., Coser, 1956; Deutsch, 1973; Sherif, 1966), there is no need to see this aspect of conflict as fundamental (see Condor & Brown, this volume). This chapter adopts a broad definition of intergroup conflict (see Hewstone & Giles, 1984), embracing studies on both social competition (achieved by defining the ingroup positively with respect to outgroups) and realistic competition over scarce resources (such as power, prestige, and wealth). While such a definition is not precise, the clarification of conflict becomes very complex when one begins to consider such factors as antecedent conditions of conflict, affective and cognitive states of the individuals involved, and stages of conflict itself (e.g., from latent to manifest; see Plon, 1975). However, this definition includes a wide range of phenomena and thus allows for a detailed examination of the present question of interest – the role of attributions, or causal explanations, in intergroup conflict.

Surprisingly, given the sustained interest in attribution theory within social psychology (see, e.g., Harvey & Weary, 1984), there has been relatively little interest in attributions at the intergroup level, although Horai (1977) has argued that differing attributions for the same set of events are critical supports for intergroup conflict. Cooper and Fazio (1979) have stated more forcefully that "one of the important bases of intergroup conflict can be found in the motivated misuse of attributional rules and that the attributions thus formed serve to further sustain and nurture the conflict" (p.149). Cooper and Fazio explicitly compared attribution theory's model of the layperson as a naive scientist, searching quasi-logically for the true causes of things, with the "outrageous logic" (p.150) of intergroup attributions. However, these authors were unable to report much relevant research and it is only in recent years that a better understanding of the relationship between attribution theory and intergroup relations has been gained.

The aim of this chapter is to demonstrate the empirical and theoretical bases of an attributional approach to intergroup conflict, by looking at the role of attributions in the development and reduction of conflict. The first part of the chapter concerns the maintenance of intergroup conflict by explanations for the behavior of ingroup and outgroup members. The motivational bases of such attributions are examined separately for members of majority/dominant and minority/dominated groups, by considering the group functions fulfilled by attributions. Cognitive bases of intergroup attribution are then examined, with a focus on the role of expectancies and schema-based attribution. The second part of the chapter explores the reduction of intergroup conflict, by investigating attributions for behavior that disconfirms expectancies. A role for attributions is also proposed in memory for such behavior, with implications for changing intergroup perceptions. This leads to an analysis of models of schema change. The chapter concludes by setting out a model of the role of attributions in intergroup conflict.

The Development and Maintenance of Intergroup Conflict

Rather than attempt to explain when, where, and how intergroup conflict begins, the attributional approach seems most valuable in underlining how conflict is supported, even exacerbated. Konečni's (1979) analysis of the role of aversive events in the development of intergroup conflict states that such events represent information that affects thoughts and attitudes concerning members of the outgroup, especially when an ingroup member perceives an aversive event to be due to the actions of another group. He reports that there are literally countless examples of aggressive behavior aimed directly at members of outgroups perceived to be responsible for the occurrence of aversive events (see Gurr, 1968). In a similar vein, Billig's (1976) account of the frustration-aggression hypothesis applied to intergroup relations argues that the crucial intervening variable that links the cause (e. g., frustration due to social deprivation) with the effect (e. g., aggression in the form of a riot) is the social interpretation of the deprivation. As Billig puts it, the theories of social causation shared by the participants in such collective behavior are very important.

Starting from a more traditional attribution theory perspective, Cooper and Fazio (1979) extend Jones and Davis' (1965) correspondent inference theory to intergroup conflict. Jones and Davis proposed a strong tendency to make more extreme dispositional attributions when the behavior of an actor directly affects the attributor (hedonic relevance; see Chaiken & Cooper, 1973) and when the behavior is seen to be intended for the attributor (personalism). Cooper and Fazio proposed that both tendencies are heightened in intergroup conflict, especially for negative actions by the outgroup, since these actions may be aimed at frustrating the aspirations of the ingroup. These simplified inferences about outgroup hostility may also enhance feelings of control, because counteraction against the outgroup appears the clear solution. Cooper and Fazio offer the interesting insight that personalism, while relatively infrequent when we function as individuals, may be more typical of intergroup encounters. The term "vicarious personalism" is introduced for one group's perception that the other group's actions are aimed specifically at them. This perception results in a more negative evaluation of the outgroup than would be implied by a dispassionate inference process; in short, "A simplistic correspondent inference about the evil nature of the outgroup is made" (p. 152). If such attribution bias and distortion of evidence is characteristic of intergroup perception, then there should be clear differences in the explanation of ingroup and outgroup members' behavior. This evidence is now reviewed.

Explanations for the Behavior of Ingroup and Outgroup Members

This section deals with how members of different social groups explain the behavior of members of their own and other social groups (Hewstone & Jaspars, 1982a, 1984). (To be more precise, explanations may refer not only to behavior, but also to the outcomes of behavior, or to the social conditions characterizing different groups.) The studies reviewed show that the causes of the same behavior can be perceived in very different ways depending on who performs the behavior.

Historically, Fauconnet (1928) was clearly aware of the impact of social categorization on attribution, writing: "People with bad reputations are accused and convicted on the basis of evidence which one would consider insufficient if an unfavorable prejudice did not relate them to the crime in advance" (translation; cited in Heider, 1944, p. 363), and Zillig (1928) demonstrated experimentally that a "bad" act is easily connected with a "bad" person. More recently, Ugwuegbu's (1979) simulated jury study using white American students reported that when the evidence for a forcible rape was marginal, a black defendant was rated significantly more culpable than was a white defendant.

The first empirical study to explore intergroup attributions was that of Taylor and Jaggi (1974), carried out in southern India against the background of conflict between Hindu and Muslim groups. The basic hypothesis of the study was that observers (Hindu adults) would make internal attributions for other Hindus (i.e., ingroup members) performing socially desirable acts, and external attributions for undesirable acts. The reverse was predicted for attributions to Muslim outgroup members (see Table 1). The predictions were clearly borne out by the data.

Table 1. Ethnocentric attributions

Type of behavior	Type of actor	
	Ingroup	Outgroup
Positive	Dispositional	Situational
Negative	Situational	Dispositional

(after Taylor & Jaggi, 1974; from Hewstone & Jaspars, 1982a)

Because of the importance of this study, a conceptual replication was carried out in Southeast Asia (Hewstone & Ward, 1985). A first study used Malay and Chinese students in Malaysia. Malays behaved as expected, by making internal attributions for the positive behaviors of their own group members, but for negative behaviors by the Chinese. This is clear ethnocentric attribution, with the effect for ingroup favoritism actually far stronger than that for outgroup denigration. Contrary to predictions, the Chinese also favored the Malay actors at the expense of their own group. A second study was then carried out in neighbouring Singapore. The Malays there retained the tendency to make internal attributions for positive behavior by their own group, but they did not make significantly different attributions for positive and negative behavior by the Chinese. The Chinese did not significantly favor either group. There are many differences between Malaysia and Singapore (see Ward & Hewstone, 1985), but these different sets of results can be seen in terms of the different levels of inter-ethnic group conflict in the two countries, with more conflict in the politically rather tense and potentially assimilationist culture of Malaysia than in relatively tolerant, multicultural Singapore. These attributional data were backed up by ethnic stereotypes. In Malaysia, Malays saw themselves in positive terms, but viewed the Chinese in predominantly negative terms (as did the Chinese themselves). The Singaporean data revealed an overall strikingly lower degree of stereotyping.

These comparative results are interesting in the light of Triandis' (1979) proposal that distortions in the attribution process are a major factor in intergroup conflict. Bond, Hewstone, Wan, & Chiu (1985) reported consistent data for intergroup attributions of sex-typed behaviors in both Hong Kong and the United States. Although both their studies found group-serving biases in the way males and females explained sex differences in behavior, the results were more robust for the American than for the Chinese respondents, a finding that was interpreted in terms of the longer history of the women's movement and more overt male-female rivalry (e.g., for equal opportunities) in the United States.

Although it should be remembered that Taylor and Jaggi's (1974) results were qualified by Hewstone and Ward (1985), Taylor and Jaggi suggested that future research might go beyond the internal-external classification of attributions to give more specific predictions concerning how ingroup and outgroup behavior would be explained. They noted particularly Weiner's (e.g., Weiner et al., 1972) model for classifying the explanations that people give for success and failure.

Weiner's work in achievement situations has emphasized four causal factors used to explain success and failure: ability, effort, task difficulty, and luck (e.g., Weiner, 1979). By considering both the antecedents and consequences of causal attributions to these four (and other) factors, Weiner has shown why it is necessary to move beyond Heider's (1958) fundamental distinction between internal and external causes. For example, the perception that an individual failed because of lack of effort has different implications than an ascription to lack of ability. Although both causes are internal, more punishment is likely when lack of effort is the explanation (Weiner & Kukla, 1970), whereas lower future expectancies of success arise from lack of ability attribution (Weiner, Nierenberg, & Goldstein, 1976). According to Weiner, the effort and ability attributions are similarly classified on a dimension of locus (both are internal), but are differently classified on a dimension of causal stability (effort is unstable, ability is stable). A third dimension, controllability, has also been introduced, because some causes identically classified on both locus and stability dimensions result in different reactions. Although there may be additional causal dimensions (e.g., intentionality, globality) and the major three dimensions do not appear orthogonal, the four main achievement attributions have received most attention; they can be classified as follows: ability (internal, stable, uncontrollable), effort (internal, unstable, controllable), luck (external, unstable, uncontrollable), task difficulty (external, stable, uncontrollable).

Using this approach one can extend Taylor and Jaggi's model of intergroup attribution and apply it to achievement situations (see Deaux & Emswiller, 1974; Greenberg & Rosenfield, 1979; Yarkin, Town, & Wallston, 1982). The ingroup-serving attributions linked to Weiner's dimensions are shown in Table 2. These possibilities broadly support Taylor and Jaggi's predictions of internal attribution for ingroup positive and outgroup negative acts, but external attribution for ingroup negative and outgroup positive acts, with one exception. Both outgroup success and ingroup failure can be attributed internally to effort, derogating the outgroup and favoring the ingroup respectively (see Ho & Lloyd, 1983). As an example of the former attribution, Pettigrew (1979) refers to "explaining away" the positive behavior of the outgroup in terms of "high motivation and effort." As an example of the latter attribution, Hewstone, Jaspars and Lalljee (1982) reported that "public" (i.e. private) schoolboys ascribed the failure of an ingroup member more to lack of effort than they did

Table 2. Ingroup-serving and outgroup-derogating attributions in achievement contexts

Type of outcome	Type of actor	
	Ingroup	Outgroup
Success	Ability (internal, stable, uncontrollable)	Effort (internal, unstable, controllable)
		Luck (external, unstable, uncontrollable)
		Task (external, stable, uncontrollable)
Failure	Luck (external, unstable, uncontrollable)	Ability (internal, stable, uncontrollable)
	Task (external, stable, uncontrollable)	
	Effort (internal, unstable, controllable)	

that of an outgroup, "comprehensive" (i.e. state) schoolboy, whose failure was ascribed to lack of ability. The "comprehensive" boys, however, explained failure of an ingroup member more in terms of bad luck than they did that of an outgroup member.

The extension of Taylor and Jaggi's (1974) work using Weiner's approach may appear somewhat limited in its focus on achievement situations, but it is also useful in drawing attention to both motivational (e.g., desire to present one's group in a positive light) and cognitive (e.g., performing in line with expectancies) underpinnings of intergroup attribution. The following two sections explore these two bases of intergroup attribution, arguing for an integration.

Motivational Bases of Intergroup Attribution

Weiner (1982; see also 1985a) wrote that attributions appear to be sufficient antecedents for the elicitation of a number of emotions, including anger, pride (self-esteem), and resignation. He also argued that the underlying dimensions of attributions were significant, and sometimes necessary, determinants of these affective reactions. To consider the emotional consequences of intergroup attributions, one has to generalize from Weiner's work; in this section the positive functions of attributions are considered separately for majority, or dominant, and minority, or dominated, groups.

Majority Groups

According to Weiner, pride and positive self-esteem are experienced as a consequence of attributing a positive outcome to the self, whereas negative self-esteem is experienced when a negative outcome is ascribed to oneself. Thus one can see what emotional consequences follow from attributing both ingroup success and outgroup failure to internal, stable causes. Interestingly, Weiner acknowledged that pride can be felt vicariously in seeing a relative, friend, or fellow countryman succeed for internal reasons, although he did not discuss "instances of affective experience mediated by personal identification" (1982, p. 191). This identification of oneself as a group member and social identification with other ingroup members is, of course, fundamental to intergroup behavior (see Turner, 1982).

According to Tajfel's (1978; Tajfel & Turner, 1979) social identity theory, individuals define themselves to a large extent in terms of their social group membership and tend to seek a positive social identity (or self-definition) in terms of group membership. This positive view of the ingroup is achieved through intergroup social comparisons focused on the establishment of positively valued distinctiveness between one's own and other groups. It is proposed that the intergroup attributional bias illustrated above may function in this way for majority group members. Tajfel's (1969) cognitive analysis of prejudice made the point that an individual's system of causes must provide, as far as possible, a positive self-image. Such a purported motivational bias is essentially a group-based equivalent of individual self-serving biases in attribution. Thus, while a tendency has been found for individuals to explain events in ways that serve their own needs by enhancing their personal identity (see, e.g., Weary, 1979; Zuckerman, 1979), group members also tend to explain events in ways that enhance their social identity. The attributional approach extends social identity theory in one important way. Tajfel (1978) held that a positive social identity was conferred by intergroup comparisons in terms of differences that favor the ingroup. However, a study of rival university groups in Hong Kong (Hewstone, Bond, & Wan, 1983) found that it was unnecessary that an intergroup difference favor the ingroup, because unwelcome aspects of reality could be avoided by attributional means (e.g., by making ingroup-serving explanations for differences that favored the outgroup). Thus intergroup attributions can sustain conflict and, as will be seen, interfere with attempts at conflict reduction.

Tajfel (1981) has also mentioned a "social explanatory" function of stereotypes, referring to the creation and maintenance of group ideologies that justify and explain intergroup relations, particularly reactions to and treatment of outgroup members (Hewstone & Giles, 1986). This explanatory function may be fulfilled by victimization (Howard, 1984) and by bizarre "causal misperception" Campbell (1967), which results in the outgroup being perceived as the cause of the ingroup's hostility (see also Ichheiser, 1949; Sartre, 1954). Scapegoating too has an attributional basis which has been referred to by many authors (e.g., Allport, 1954; Bains, 1983; Fauconnet, 1928; Heider, 1944; LeVine & Campbell, 1972). At a societal level, group-based attributions underlie the "conspiracy theory," whereby the ills of contemporary society are attributed to the "conscious machinations of a few individuals" (Billig, 1978, p.317). As Billig reports, the conspiracy theory provides simple, "personal" attributions for complex, social events, by tracing events to a small but easily identifiable outgroup, such as, at different points in history, witches, Jews, Jesuits, freemasons, and Marxists (see Poliakov, 1980).

Minority Groups

Just as for majority groups, causal attributions can be related to group-esteem for minority groups. However, a more interesting emotional consequence is, perhaps, anger, as experienced when a negative, self-related outcome or event is attributed to factors controllable by others (Weiner, 1982). For minority groups, an attributional approach can contribute to the neglected analysis of the experience of discrimination (e.g., Griffin, 1961; Mazrui, 1980). Experimental work by Dion and colleagues (Dion & Earn, 1975; Dion, Earn, & Yee, 1978) has shown exactly this attribution-emotion link. Lone minority group members (e.g., Jews) who attributed their failure in a group ticket-passing task to religious discrimination by gentiles, reported feeling more aggression, sadness, anxiety, and egotism on the Mood Adjective Check List than did subjects who had not made such attributions.

Another important type of attribution for minority group members is "system blame" (see Geber & Newman, 1980; Myrdal, 1944; Taylor & Walsh, 1979), as in black people's explanations for what might appear to be personal failures (in the eyes of whites). Hewstone and Jaspars (1982b) examined the explanations for institutionalized racial discrimination given by young blacks and whites in Britain. Black respondents generally attributed the phenomena of discrimination more to white members of the system, and less to personal characteristics of blacks, than did white respondents, a tendency that was polarized in group discussion. Simmons (1978) wrote that this system blame may be a very important reaction to life in a racist society, because it protects self-esteem. In a similar vein, Gurin, Gurin, Lao, and Beattie (1969) reported young blacks in the United States who felt that economic or discriminatory factors were more important than individuall skill and personal qualities in explaining the problems they faced. At one level these young people might seem to have an external locus of control, a belief that rewards are not controlled by themselves (see Rotter, 1966). It has usually been assumed that internal locus of control represents a positive orientation, but Gurin et al. suggest that this is not so for people disadvantaged by minority status, for whom an internal locus might lead to self- (and ingroup) derogation and blame. Gurin et al. showed that those young blacks who blamed the system often aspired to jobs that were nontraditional for blacks, and they were more ready to engage in collective action.

From the above considerations, an attributional approach can illuminate the important question of the extent to which 'domination-recognition' conflicts can be paths to social change (Apfelbaum & Lubek, 1976). Attributions would appear to play an important role in generating what Billig (1976) called an "ideology of discontent," whereby a powerful outgroup is perceived to be the cause of, e.g., racial discrimination (Caplan & Paige, 1968) and the dominant group develops a positive ingroup ideology and challenges the dominant group. Tajfel and Turner (1979) maintain that low status groups only challenge high status groups if they perceive the status relationship as illegitimate and unstable (see Turner & Brown, 1978). It is therefore interesting to note reported relationships between ingroup-serving attributions and measures of perceived illegitimacy and instability for minority groups (see Bond et al., 1985; Hewstone et al., 1983). However, it is still not clear whether attributions play the important causal role of determining such perceptions and, in turn, conflict, or whether they are reflections of developing intergroup conflict. Future work should therefore analyze the role of intergroup attributions in more detail, using correlational and causal modeling techniques.

A possible mediational role for attributions should also be considered in cases of "asymmetrical" social perception, where members of minority groups evaluate themselves negatively and a dominant group positively (Schwarzwald & Yinon, 1977). Demonstrations of such attributional "self-hate" (Lewin, 1948) have been reported for women (see Deaux, 1984; but cf. Feldman-Summers & Kiesler, 1974) and for ethnic Chinese in Malaysia (Hewstone & Ward, 1985). In this relatively rare case, attributions are dysfunctional for the ingroup, with emotions of helplessness and resignation engendered by the attribution of negative outcomes to internal, stable factors (Weiner, 1982).

Cognitive Bases of Intergroup Conflict

Expectancy-Based Attributions

Just as Weiner's work led to a consideration of motivational bases of inter-group attribution, so too it leads to a discussion of cognitive factors. Weiner et al. (1972) reported that attributions were made to stable and internal causes when there was a fit between expectancy and performance, while a performance discrepant with expectancies was attributed to unstable causes. Consistent with this view, Regan, Straus, and Fazio (1974) found that behavior in line with one's expectations of another was attributed to dispositional qualities of the actor, whereas behavior discrepant with expectations was attributed to a situational factor. (The explanation of inconsistent behavior is treated in detail below.) At the level of self-attribution, Miller and Ross (1975) have also argued that the self-enhancing attribution bias (the tendency to take credit for success) can be explained by cognitive factors, including expectancy. People may expect to succeed and therefore accept more responsibility for success as this outcome fits with expectations.

At an intergroup level, Deaux (1976, 1984) has linked causal attributions (for the performance of males and females) to observers' initial expectations concerning performance. Thus a male's successful performance on a male-linked task was attributed more to ability than was a female's successful performance, by both male and female subjects (Deaux & Emswiller, 1974). Deaux suggested that expectancies for specific tasks could be understood in terms of more general stereotypes and she reported some evidence that general attitudes towards women and men are correlated with attributions (see Garland & Price, 1977).

Schema-Based Attributions

Following Deaux's (1976) work, cognitive social psychologists (e.g., Hamilton, 1979) began to think of stereotypes as "structural frameworks" or "schemata" in terms of which information is processed. A schema has been defined as "a cognitive structure that represents organized knowledge about a given concept or type of stimulus" (Fiske & Taylor, 1984, p.140). This knowledge structure has implications for social information processing, including perception, memory, and inference. In explaining schema-consistent or expectancy-confirming behavior, perceivers may simply rely on dispositions implied by the stereotype, not even bothering to consider additional factors (Pyszczynski & Greenberg, 1981). Given that schema-based social information processing is fast and relatively efficient, one can think of expectancy-confirming attributions as following a strategy of "minimum causation" (Shaklee & Fischhoff, 1979, cited in Shaver, 1981), whereby the search for possible causes of an effect is terminated once an effect has been adequately explained (see Pryor & Kriss, 1977; Smith & Miller, 1979). Thus Jones and Davis (1965) argued that "the perceiver's explanation comes to a stop when an intention or motive has the quality of being reason enough" (p. 220). Expectancy-confirming attributions can also be thought of in terms of the distinction between "perceived causality" (the natural cognitive unity of "actor and act"; Heider, 1944; Jones, 1979) and "higher order causal inferences" (relatively abstract judgements about the probable cause of an act; see Johnson, Jemmott, & Pettigrew, 1984; Weary, Rich, Harvey, & Ickes, 1980).

Salience Effects

Taylor and Fiske (1978) have considered this dual system in detail, proposing a dichotomy between "automatic" and "controlled" processing. They integrate evidence from a number of empirical studies to propose that many perceivers seek a single, sufficient, and salient explanation for behavior, and that causal attributions are often shaped by highly salient stimuli. Both Heider (1944) and Michotte (1946) demonstrated that perception of causality was heavily influenced by strong, vivid stimuli, and Taylor and Fiske extend this view to more social forms of perception. Their overall hypothesis is that attention determines what information is salient, and that perceptually salient information is overrepresented in subsequent causal explanations. For example, a single black person in a small group of otherwise white people should be salient to observers and also perceived as disproportionately causal in the group's performance (Taylor, Fiske, Etcoff, & Ruderman, 1978). That "solo" person's race is the basis for his or her distinctiveness, and that attribute will be highly available (Tversky & Kahneman, 1974) as an explanation for the solo black person's behavior. Campbell (1967) also noted that salience can lead to erroneous causal attribution, referring to the fact that multiple, diffuse, and complex stimuli representing environmental factors (e.g., the social conditions of some minority groups) may be overlooked in favor of salient stimuli (such as skin colour). Given that attention to these salient stimuli also leads perceivers to mistake members of a different group for each other (Malpass & Kravitz, 1969; Taylor et al., 1978), it is easy to envisage how outgroup members are assumed to be similar to one another and, in turn, how that similarity may be used as a basis for causal reasoning (Read, 1983, 1984).

Although salience effects are intuitively plausible and empirically demonstrable, there remain problems with this interpretation of intergroup attribution. For example, in different studies a novel or salient person's behavior has been viewed both more and less situationally than that of a nonsalient person (McArthur & Post, 1977). In addition, if Taylor and Fiske (1978) propose that causal agents are seen as efficacious in proportion to their perceptual salience, then why are outgroup members not given more credit for success? Such cognitive factors may be especially important in controlled laboratory conditions, but their importance in situations of conflict would seem to be secondary to both motivational factors and other cognitive factors such as expectancies.

Confirmatory Bias

Returning to the role of expectancies, attributions appear to intrude into other cognitive biases which tend to confirm behavioral expectancies, and could help to maintain conflict. An example of such a bias is the tendency towards hypothesis confirmation shown by perceivers asked to test a hypothesis about another person (Snyder, 1981, 1984). Stereotypes generate expectancies and people seem to feel more confident when confirming their hypotheses than when using information to disconfirm an alternative explanation (Hansen, 1980). In fact, research suggests that individuals regard confirming evidence as more convincing and probative, as well as more relevant and informative, than disconfirming evidence (see Alloy & Tabachnik, 1984).

Snyder's (1981, 1984) work also shows how stereotypes are used to constrain the behavioral alternatives of others, and to engender stereotype-confirming behavior from others (e.g., Snyder, Tanke, & Berscheid, 1977; Word, Zanna, & Cooper, 1974). Attributions seem to influence whether such behavioral confirmation perseveres beyond the specific context in which it occurs (Snyder, 1984). Perseveration seems more likely when the perceiver is led to attribute behavioral confirmation to underlying traits and dispositions of the actor. For example, consider an ingroup member who interacts with a member of a perceived hostile outgroup. Acting upon these beliefs, the outgroup member is treated as hostile and then actually behaves in a manner consistent with this label. If the ingroup member is led to believe that this hostile behavior reflects corresponding personality dispositions, then his or her behavioral confirmation strategy will extend to further outgroup members (see Cooper & Fazio, 1979; Snyder & Swann, 1978).

The outcome of confirmatory hypothesis testing is that expectancies are confirmed, in the form of self-fulfilling prophecies (see also Darley & Fazio, 1980). As Snyder put it, "Social beliefs can and do create their own social reality" (1984, p. 193). Cooper and Fazio (1979) contend that such self-fulfilling prophecies are even more likely to occur in intergroup interaction; because groups are almost never totally homogeneous, consisting of a distribution of individuals with certain traits, it becomes more likely that some evidence can be found to support one's preconceptions.

An Integration

In view of the foregoing discussion of motivational and cognitive factors in intergroup attribution, an integration seems most plausible. Attribution theorists (e.g., Bradley, 1978; Miller & Ross, 1975) have discussed this issue in some detail, leading Tetlock and Levi (1982) to conclude that for the present it appears impossible to choose between the two viewpoints. Similarly, Turner (1981), in the area of intergroup relations, has argued that cognitive (social categorization) and motivational (social comparison) processes have complementary effects on intergroup differentiation. Under laboratory conditions, and with minimal groups, cognitive factors may well be sufficient for intergroup attribution, while Greenberg and Rosenfield (1979) have argued that ethnocentric attribution in the absence of expectancies must reflect a motivational bias.[1] Perhaps the more important implication for studies of intergroup conflict is that such a variety of potential cognitive and motivational bases of intergroup attribution exist. This fact further underlines the importance of the phenomenon, particularly when outgroup behavior actually disconfirms expectations and thus has the potential to reduce conflict by changing intergroup perceptions. This topic is considered in the remainder of the present chapter.

Behavior That Disconfirms Expectations: Implications for the Reduction of Intergroup Conflict

Notwithstanding the importance of expectancies, and tendencies towards expectancy confirmation, it should be emphasized that perceivers are not always led blindly to ignore actual behavior in favor of expectancies. Alloy and Tabachnik's (1984) review of human covariation jugments refers to the prevalent view that preconceived notions (e. g., expectations, stereotypes, schemata) distort the accurate assessment of event covariation (see, e. g., Crocker, 1981; Nisbett & Ross, 1980). They emphasize, however, that people's judgment of covariation is influenced by situational information in the form of true-event covariation, and not only in the absence of expectations. A particularly important issue for the reduction of intergroup conflict is how perceivers react to situational information about the outgroup that disconfirms their negative expectations. For example, the "contact hypothesis" – the belief that positive association with persons from a disliked outgroup will lead to the growth of liking and respect for that group (Cook, 1978) – appears to be based, in part at least, on the value of disconfirming negative expectancies about the outgroup. An attributional analysis of contact research points clearly to some of its pitfalls: researchers must ensure that counterstereotypic behavior cannot be "explained away" in terms of situational demands or individual exceptions to the rule (Hewstone & Brown, 1986; Pettigrew, 1979; Williams, 1964).[2] How then is unexpected behavior explained, and what implications does this have for the reduction of intergroup conflict?

---

1 Unfortunately, it is not possible to rule out the role of expectations in Greenberg and Rosenfield's (1979) study. An extrasensory perception task was chosen from pilot work as one on which no race-based (black-white) expectations existed, but it remains possible that highly ethnocentric subjects (the only subjects who showed intergroup attributional bias) believed blacks to be inferior on this task.

2 Attributional approaches to many other forms of conflict reduction could be or have been put forward: e. g., intergroup cooperation that results in failure (Worchel & Norvell, 1980); attitude change by forced compliance (Cooper & Fazio, 1979); alteration of intergroup perceptions based on the actor-observer hypothesis (Rose, 1981); education in situational causality (McArthur, 1982; but see Johnson et al., 1984); and positive discrimination (Garcia, Erskine, Hawn, & Casmay, 1981; Linville & Jones, 1980).

Attributions for Behavior That Disconfirms Expectancies

Presentation of information that disconfirms expectancies has the significant consequence that it appears especially to promote spontaneous attributional thinking (Weiner, 1985b). In different studies it has been shown that attribution-relevant information was most sought when prior expectancies were disconfirmed (Pyszczynski & Greenberg, 1981; Wong & Weiner, 1981) and that an incongruent act was more likely to elicit an explanation as a story continuation than was a congruent act (Hastie, 1984). As Hastie points out, these findings are consistent with some philosophical analyses of the perception of causation (e.g., Hart & Honoré, 1959; Mackie, 1974) which have emphasized the importance of unexpectedness as a condition for causal reasoning.

The question that follows is, what type of explanation is given for unexpected behavior? Kulik (1983) presents evidence for the role played by causal attribution processes in belief perseverance. He reports that perception of the causal importance of situational factors was influenced by the degree to which an observed behavior was consistent with prior beliefs about the actor. Behavior that was consistent with prior conceptions was attributed to dispositional characteristics of the actor. Furthermore, situational factors that would in other cases be seen as compelling explanations were ignored in favor of dispositional factors as causes of expected behavior (see pp. 55–56 above). In contrast, inconsistent behavior was apt to be situationally attributed. Even settings normally considered to inhibit the observed behavior were judged instead as causal. Kulik (1983) points out that this confirmatory attributional tendency allows the perceiver to dismiss the potential belief-altering implications of out-of-role behavior (Jones & Davis, 1965) and can thus be seen as a factor that impedes the reduction of intergroup conflict.

Alloy and Tabachnik (1984) also propose that perceivers, by attributing behavior that disconfirms their expectancies to unstable or external factors, arm themselves against the detection of covariation that might change their beliefs (e.g., Bell, Wicklund, Manko, & Larkin, 1976; Deaux, 1976; Hayden & Mischel, 1976; Zadny & Gerard, 1974). Such a simple process would act to preserve and protect stereotypes about the outgroup. Because stereotypes refer to perceivers' assumptions about the dispositional attributes of ingroup and outgroup members, any behavior violating the stereotype could be avoided on the basis that it reflected situational influences and thus did not derive from the personal characteristics of the actor (Cooper & Fazio, 1979; Hamilton, 1979; Stephan & Rosenfield, 1982). As Merton argued, "the systematic condemnation of the out-grouper continues largely irrespective of what he does" (1957, p. 428).

Memory for Unexpected Behavior

It might also be hoped that unexpected behavior would effect change of inter-group beliefs by being favored in memory. The available literature suggests, however, that this effect is unlikely, and again attributions are important. One set of experimental evidence reports a tendency to overrecall expectation-consistent instances relative to inconsistent instances, as well as a tendency to "in-trude" expectancy-consistent instances that were never actually observed (e. g., Cantor & Mischel, 1977; Woll & Yopp, 1978). In contrast, more recent work on social memory has pointed to the relatively high recall of unexpected or incongruent information (e. g., Crocker, Hannah, & Weber, 1983; Hastie & Kumar, 1979), subject to certain qualifications concerning time pressure and memory load (Srull, 1981). Both Crocker et al. (1983) and Hastie (1984) pointed to the role of attributions in the recall of incongruent information.

Crocker et al. (1983) suggested that the cognitive activity involved in trying to generate an attribution for incongruent behavior may make the incongruent item easier to recall (Hastie & Kumar, 1979), although Wells (1982) reported that the explicit making of an attribution only produced good memory for event infor-mation if the causal information led to an unambiguous implication of causal lo-cus (e. g., clearly person or situation attribution). Crocker et al. further proposed that the type of causal attribution that is provided for an act will determine whether or not the act is well remembered. Their research showed that an unex-pected act would be most likely to be recalled only if it was explained with refer-ence to the actor's dispositions. On the other hand, if the behavior was attributed to a situational cause, it was equally likely to be recalled whether it was congru-ent or incongruent. Correlational analyses indicated that impressions of the ac-tor were mediated by causal attributions: there was a moderate positive correla-tion between recall and impressions when an item was attributed to a dispositional cause ($r = 0.27$), but there was no relationship between recall and impressions when the item was attributed to a situational cause ($r = 0.08$).

Hastie's (1984) results also imply that causal reasoning instigated by the oc-currence of an unexpected event is one determinant of the subsequent superior recall of that event. It should be noted, however, that Hastie identifies it as an important part of his paradigm that subjects were asked to form an impression of a target person by integrating all available information (and not discounting some of it). Arguably, in many situations of intergroup conflict, ingroup mem-bers would discount or "explain away" positive behaviors associated with out-group members (Pettigrew, 1979).

It might appear from the literature on attribution and memory for unex-pected behavior that belief change will be brought about by providing incon-gruent behavior linked with a dispositional attribution. Such a conclusion would be both naive and premature. One of the clearest lessons to emerge from the study of intergroup contact is that the experience of positive contact rarely generalizes to other outgroup members, because of the cognitive processes (in-cluding causal attribution) that classify the single outgroup member as a "spe-cial case" and thus prevent belief change (see Allport's, 1954, "re-fencing device"; Williams', 1964, "exemption mechanism"). Crocker et al. (1983) suggest that, in the absence of a dispositional attribution, people may conclude that incongruent behavior does not provide good evidence of the actor's typical behavior. In situations of intergroup contact, what is so often missing is information that leads the participants to view their partners as typical outgroup members, and thus to prevent them from explaining away positive behavior of the outgroup member (Hewstone & Brown, 1986).

Models of Schema Change

Crocker, Fiske, and Taylor (1984) argue that one of the main ways that schemata can change is through exposure to incongruent information (i.e., information that is improbable, given the schema). Although this view supports the present chapter's concern with attributions for behavior that disconfirms expectancies, it should not be assumed that a single item of incongruent information will have much impact on a well-developed schema with large quantities of schema-congruent information. The reduction of intergroup conflict will almost always require intervention of a longitudinal nature, whose effects can work cumulatively (see Pettigrew, 1986; Sherif, 1979).

Weber and Crocker (1983) have compared three models of stereotype or schema change in response to new information. The "bookkeeping" model (Rothbart, 1981) views stereotype change as a gradual process in which each new instance of stereotype-discrepant information modifies the existing stereotype. Any single piece of disconfirming evidence elicits only a minor change; substantial changes occur incrementally with the accumulation of evidence that disconfirms the stereotypes. The "conversion" model (Rothbart, 1981) is more dramatic, allowing for a single, salient incongruent instance to bring about schema change. According to this second model, schema change is all-or-none and is not engendered by minor disconfirmations. Evidence for this model is provided by Gurwitz and Dodge (1977), who reported that stereotype change was greater when disconfirming evidence was concentrated in one person's description, than when it was dispersed across three people (each of whom only partly disconfirmed the stereotype). (The opposite was true for confirming evidence, where the dispersed pattern of information led to greater stereotypic responding than did the concentrated pattern.) Similarly, Rose (1981) argued that intergroup contact in the form of an intimate relationship with a single outgroup member is a powerful method of stereotype change, because it offers the possibility of multiple disconfirmations of the stereotype. The third model, "subtyping," views stereotypes as hierarchical structures that evolve through experience (Ashmore, 1981; Brewer, Dull, & Lui, 1981; Taylor, 1981). According to this model, when all the disconfirming evidence is concentrated within a few individuals, those individuals will be subtyped (seen as a separate subcategory), and they will be seen as "exceptions that prove the rule." The subtyping model predicts more change when incongruent information is dispersed across individuals than when it is concentrated in a few.

Which model is supported by the available evidence? Weber and Crocker's (1983) four studies provide partial support for two of the models. They contend that the subtyping model may be the best description of stereotype change when incongruent information is concentrated in a few individuals – the small number of individuals in whom information is concentrated are easily sub-typed. (Weber and Crocker explain this contradiction of Gurwitz and Dodge's [1977] finding by suggesting that the use of sorority groups in the earlier study may have ruled out perception of differences between group members.) The bookkeeping model, however, may describe how stereotypes change when incongruent information is dispersed across a larger number of individuals (because in this condition individuals could not be easily subtyped, and the stereotype changes with each new piece of incongruent information). In addition, Weber and Crocker acknowledge that the conversion model might apply when a perceiver is unsure of a stereotype, and hence easily swayed by available information.

An attributional analysis of this research provides some illumination. It would argue, first, that both the bookkeeping and, especially, the conversion models run the risk that discrepant information will be explained away. Attributing discrepant information to, for example, some special personal characteristic of the actor implies that studies of intimate contact (e.g., Rose, 1981) will generalize across situations, but not across other outgroup members. As Hewstone and Brown (1986) have argued, this failure to generalize attitude change is one of the central weaknesses of the traditional contact hypothesis. Interestingly, Gurwitz and Dodge (1977) explain their finding, of stereotype change when disconfirming evidence was concentrated, in quasi-attributional terms. They suggest that it may be relatively easy to discount disconfirming behaviors when each person is described as demonstrating just one of then, but that when one individual's behavior is completely discrepant with the stereotype, disconfirming evidence is too salient to be discounted. This explanation is ironic, because the authors ignore the possibility that subjects discount the evidence as relevant to outgroup members in general. As Weber and Crocker (1983) note, it was apparently more difficult for subjects to dismiss instances as "exceptions" when the information was dispersed across group members. Most important, Weber and Crocker found that people's stereotypes about these (occupational) groups changed most when they were presented with counterstereotypical information about representative members of those groups. The same information, when associated with atypical members of the category in question, had much less effect in modifying attitudes. However, even representative members tended to be subtyped from the rest of the group, supporting the subtyping model's prediction that "members who strongly disconfirm the group's stereotype are viewed as unrepresentative of the overall group and are subtyped" (Weber & Crocker, 1983, p.973).

The above discussion reveals the value of an atributional analysis of schema change, but also cautions against hasty conclusions about the extent to which schemata can be changed. We know that stereotypes are not applied to every individual outgroup member (see Locksley, Borgida, Brekke, & Hepburn, 1980;

Locksley, Hepburn & Ortiz, 1982), but experience with an atypical outgroup member need have no implications for schema change, unless we can be sure that the relevant schema has been "activated" (Crocker et al., 1984). Many interventions aimed at reducing intergroup conflict, such as programs of intergroup contact, may fail for the very simple reason that the schema activated is a rather specific one (e. g., well-educated blacks) and not the negative schema of outgroup members in general that underpins the conflict. Under these conditions the behavior of atypical outgroup members can be explained in such a way that the incongruent information has no impact at all on intergroup conflict.

The Role of Attributions in Intergroup Conflict: A Model

The role of attributions in intergroup conflict can be summarized in a model (see Fig. 1) based on, but extending, previous work (Cooper & Fazio, 1979; Deaux, 1976; Hewstone & Brown, 1986; Stephan & Rosenfield, 1982; Taylor & Jaggi, 1974). This model draws together all the work reviewed in this chapter concerning the development, maintenance and attempts at the reduction of conflict.

Vicarious personalism sets the scene for sustained intergroup conflict, because ingroup members perceive that the outgroup's actions are aimed at and intended for them. This perception results in an extremely hostile view of the outgroup, a view that generates negative expectancies for outgroup behavior which can be confirmed by one of two routes. First, outgroup behavior may be perceived to confirm expectancies and is thus attributed internally (to stable causes), maintaining conflict. Second, negative expectancies for outgroup behavior may lead to modifications of the behavior of ingroup members, outgroup behavior that is affected by the ingroup's expectancies, and outgroup behavior that actually confirms ingroup expectancies (a self-fulfilling prophecy). This behavior is again attributed internally, maintaining conflict.

The model also allows for outgroup behavior that does, or is perceived to, disconfirm expectancies, and that generates attributional activity. Unexpected behavior can be explained in various ways. First, it can be attributed to external factors, which again maintains conflict. Alternatively, the unexpected behavior can be attributed internally, with different consequences depending on how the individual outgrouper is perceived. If perceived as atypical, the behavior can be "explained away," by treating the individual as a "special case." This attribution means that the behavior has little impact on the outgroup stereotype. If the individual is seen as a typical outgroup member, then there is a real chance of generalized change of outgroup attitudes, although this potentially conflict-reducing change may still be diluted by subtyping.

Such a model helps to explain why intergroup conflict often persists despite information that disconfirms negative expectancies concerning the outgroup, and despite programs aimed at conflict reduction: because in two out of three cases where outgroup behavior is perceived to disconfirm expectancies, con-

Fig. 1. The role of attributions in the continuation or reduction of intergroup conflict

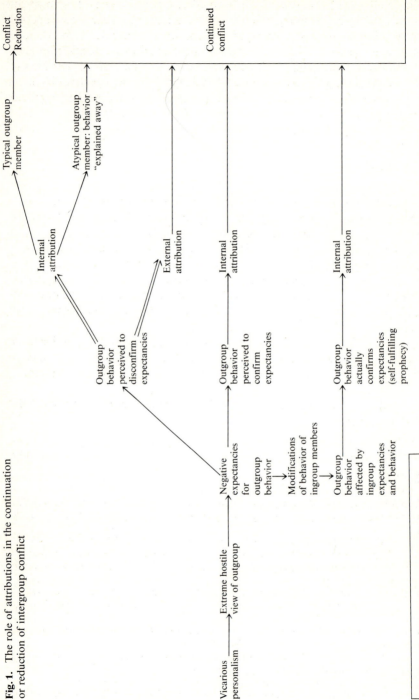

Note: ⟹ denotes increased attributional activity.

flict-sustaining attributions can be offered. This model could be further tested by process analysis, including reaction time studies (does it take longer to explain behavior that disconfirms negative outgroup expectancies?) and correlations between variables (e.g., is there a significant positive correlation between outgroup expectancies and type of attribution?). Such analysis should help to build a more general model (see Fiske & Taylor, 1984, chap. 10) and, if necessary, to specify the nature and causal order of types of attribution (Smith & Miller, 1983).

Conclusion

Some researchers have claimed that the emphasis on attribution processes in recent social psychology is exaggerated (e.g., Manis, 1977). This view cannot be stated accurately with regard to intergroup attributions, where the available evidence is still quite modest (for reviews see Hewstone & Jaspars, 1982a, 1984; Wilder & Cooper, 1981). The present chapter is another attempt to redress the balance in favor of intrapersonal and interpersonal work in this field. It has attempted to specify a role for attributions at various stages of intergroup conflict, but without exaggerating the role of attributions or denying the relevance of many other processes.

It is hoped that by attempting to specify the role of attributions in this manner, and by detailing their importance for both the maintenance and reduction of intergroup conflict, more work will be devoted to this topic in the future.

Acknowledgment. I am grateful to Howard Giles for his comments on an earlier draft of this chapter.

References

Alloy, L. B., & Tabachnik, N. (1984). Assessment of covariation by humans and animals: The joint influence of prior expectations and current situational information. *Psychological Review, 91,* 112–149.

Allport, G. W. (1979). *The nature of prejudice,* 2nd ed. Reading, MA: Addison-Wesley.

Apfelbaum, E., & Lubek, I. (1976). Resolution versus revolution? The theory of conflicts in question. In L. H. Strickland, F. E. Aboud, & K. J. Gergen (Eds.), *Social psychology in transition.* New York: Plenum.

Ashmore, R. D. (1981). Sex stereotypes and implicit personality theory. In D. L. Hamilton (Ed.), *Cognitive processes in stereotyping and intergroup behavior.* Hillsdale, NJ: Erlbaum.

Bains, G. (1983). Explanations and the need for control. In M. Hewstone (Ed.), *Attribution theory: Social and functional extensions.* Oxford: Blackwell.

Bell, L. G., Wicklund, R. A., Manko, G., & Larkin, C. (1976). When unexpected behavior is attributed to the environment. *Journal of Research in Personality, 10,* 316–327.

Billig, M. (1976). *Social psychology and intergroup relations.* London: Academic.

Billig, M. (1978). *Fascists: A social psychological view of the National Front.* London: Harcourt Brace Jovanovitch.

Bond, M.H., Hewstone, M., Wan, K.-C., & Chiu, C.-K. (1985). Group-serving attributions across intergroup contexts: Cultural differences in the explanation of sex-typed behaviours. *European Journal of Social Psychology, 15,* 435–451.

Bradley, C.W. (1978). Self-serving biases in the attribution process: A re-examination of the fact or fiction question. *Journal of Personality and Social Psychology, 35,* 56–71.

Brewer, M.B., Dull, V., & Lui, L. (1981). Perceptions of the elderly: Stereotypes as prototypes. *Journal of Personality and Social Psychology, 41,* 656–670.

Campbell, D.T. (1967). Stereotypes and the perception of group differences. *American Psychologist, 22,* 817–829.

Cantor, N., & Mischel, W. (1977). Traits as prototypes: Effects on recognition memory. *Journal of Personality and Social Psychology, 35,* 38–48.

Caplan, N., & Paige, J. (1968). A study of ghetto rioters. *Scientific American, 219,* 15–21.

Chaiken, A.L., & Cooper, J. (1973). Evaluation as a function of correspondence and hedonic relevance. *Journal of Experimental Social Psychology, 9,* 257–264.

Cook, S.W. (1978). Interpersonal and attitudinal outcomes in co-operating inter-racial groups. *Journal of Research and Development in Education, 12,* 97–113.

Cooper, J., & Fazio, R.H. (1979). The formation and persistence of attitudes that support intergroup conflict. In W.G. Austin & S. Worchel (Eds.), *The social psychology of intergroup relations.* Monterey, CA: Brooks/Cole.

Coser, L.A. (1956). *The functions of social conflict.* Glencoe, IL: Free Press.

Crocker, J. (1981). Judgment of covariation by social perceivers. *Psychological Bulletin, 90,* 272–292.

Crocker, J., Fiske, S.T., & Taylor, S.E. (1984). Schematic bases of belief change. In J.R. Eiser (Ed.), *Attitudinal judgment.* New York, Springer.

Crocker, J., Hannah, D.B., & Weber, R. (1983). Person memory and causal attributions. *Journal of Personality and Social Psychology, 44,* 55–66.

Darley, J.M., & Fazio, R.H. (1980). Expectancy confirmation processes in the social interaction sequence. *American Psychologist, 35,* 867–881.

Deaux, K. (1976). Sex: A perspective on the attribution process. In J.H. Harvey, W.J. Ickes, R.F. Kidd (Eds.), *New Directions in attribution research* (Vol. 1), Hillsdale, NJ: Erlbaum.

Deaux, K. (1984). From individual differences to social categories: Analysis of a decade's research on gender. *American Psychologist, 39,* 105–116.

Deaux, K., & Emswiller, T. (1974). Explanations of successful performance on sex-linked tasks: What is skill for the male is luck for the female. *Journal of Personality and Social Psychology, 29,* 80–85.

Deutsch, M. (1973). *The resolution of conflict.* New Haven: Yale University Press.

Dion, K.L., & Earn, B.M. (1975). The phenomenology of being a target of prejudice. *Journal of Personality and Social Psychology, 32,* 944–950.

Dion, K.L., Earn, B.M., & Yee, P.H.N. (1978). The experience of being a victim of prejudice: An experimental approach. *International Journal of Psychology, 13,* 197–214.

Fauconnet, P. (1928). *La responsabilité.* Paris: Alcan.

Feldman-Summers, S., & Kiesler, S.B. (1974). Those who are number two try harder: The effect of sex on attributions of causality. *Journal of Personality and Social Psychology, 30,* 846–855.

Fiske, S.T., & Taylor, S.E. (1984). *Social cognition.* New York: Random House.

Garcia, L.T., Erskine, N., Hawn, K., & Casmay, S.R. (1981). The effect of affirmative action on attributions about minority group members. *Journal of Personality, 49,* 427–437.

Garland, H., & Price, K.H. (1977). Attitudes toward women in management and attributions for their success and failure in a managerial position. *Journal of Applied Psychology, 62,* 29–33.

Geber, B.A., & Newman, S.P. (1980). *Soweto's children: The development of attitudes.* London: Academic.

Greenberg, J., & Rosenfield, D. (1979). Whites ethnocentrism and their attributions for the behaviour of blacks: A motivational bias. *Journal of Personality, 47,* 643–657.

Griffin, J.H. (1961). *Black like me.* New York: Signet.

Gurin, P., Gurin, G., Lao, R., & Beattie, H. (1969). Internal-external control in the motivation-al dynamics of negro youth. *Journal of Social Issues, 25,* 29-53.

Gurr, T. R. (1968). Psychological factors in civil violence. *World Politics, 20,* 245-278.

Gurwitz, S. B., & Dodge, K. A. (1977). Effects of confirmations and disconfirmations on stereo-type-based attributions. *Journal of Personality and Social Psychology, 35,* 495-500.

Hamilton, D. L. (1979). A cognitive-attributional analysis of stereotyping. In L. Berkowitz (Ed.), *Advances in experimental social psychology* (Vol. 12). New York: Academic.

Hansen, R. D. (1980). Commonsense attribution. *Journal of Personality and Social Psychology, 39,* 996-1009.

Hart, H. L. A., & Honoré, A. M. (1959). *Causation in the law.* Oxford: Clarendon.

Harvey, J. H., & Weary, G. (1984). Current issues in attribution theory and research. *Annual Review of Psychology, 35,* 427-459.

Hastie, R. (1984). Causes and effects of causal attribution. *Journal of Personality and Social Psychology, 46,* 44-56.

Hastie, R., & Kumar, P. A. (1979). Person memory: Personality traits as organizing principles in memory for behaviors. *Journal of Personality and Social Psychology, 37,* 25-38.

Hayden, T., & Mischel, W. (1976). Maintaining trait consistency in the resolution of behavioral inconsistency: The wolf in sheep's clothing?. *Journal of Personality, 44,* 109-132.

Heider, F. (1944). Social perception and phenomenal causality. *Psychological Review, 51,* 358-374.

Heider, F. (1958). *The psychology of interpersonal relations.* New York: Wiley.

Hewstone, M., Bond, M. H., & Wan, K.-C. (1983). Social facts and social attributions: The ex-planation of intergroup differences in Hong Kong. *Social Cognition, 2,* 140-155.

Hewstone, M., & Brown, R. J. (1986). Contact is not enough: An intergroup perspective on the "contact hypothesis" in M. Hewstone & R. J. Brown (Eds.), *Contact and Conflict in inter-group encounters.* Oxford: Blackwell.

Hewstone, M., & Giles, H. (1984). Intergroup conflict. In A. Gale & A. J. Chapman (Eds.), *Psy-chology and social problems.* Chichester: Wiley.

Hewstone, M., & Giles, H. (1986). Social groups and social stereotypes in intergroup commu-nication. In W. B. Gudykunst (Ed.), *Intergroup communication.* London: Edward Arnold.

Hewstone, M., & Jaspars, J. (1982a). Intergroup relations and attribution processes. In H. Taj-fel (Ed.). *Social identity and intergroup relations.* Cambridge/Paris: Cambridge University Press/Maison des Sciences de l'Homme.

Hewstone, M., & Jaspars, J. (1982b). Explanations for racial discrimination: The effect of group discussion on intergroup attributions. *European Journal of Social Psychology, 12,* 1-16.

Hewstone, M., & Jaspars, J. (1984). Social dimensions of attribution. In H. Tajfel (Ed.). *The so-cial dimension: European developments in social psychology.* Cambridge/Paris: Cambridge University Press/Maison des Sciences de l'Homme.

Hewstone, M., Jaspars, J., & Lalljee, M. (1982). Social representations, social attribution and social identity: The intergroup images of "public" and "comprehensive" schoolboys. *Euro-pean Journal of Social Psychology, 12,* 241-269.

Hewstone, M., & Ward, C. (1985). Ethnocentrism and causal attribution in Southeast Asia. *Journal of Personality and Social Psychology, 48,* 614-623.

Ho, R., & Lloyd, J. I. (1983). Intergroup attribution: The role of social categories in causal at-tribution for behaviour. *Australian Journal of Psychology, 35,* 49-59.

Horai, J. (1977). Attributional conflict. *Journal of Social Issues, 33,* 88-100.

Howard, J. A. (1984). Societal influences on attribution: Blaming some victims more than oth-ers. *Journal of Personality and Social Psychology, 47,* 494-505.

Ichheiser, G. (1949). Misunderstandings in human relations: A study of false social percep-tion. *American Journal of Sociology, 55,* 1-70.

Johnson, J. T., Jemmott, J. B., & Pettigrew, T. F. (1984). Causal attribution and dispositional in-ference: Evidence of inconsistent judgments. *Journal of Experimental Social Psychology, 20,* 567-585.

Jones, E. E. (1979). The rocky road from acts to dispositions, *American Psychologist, 34,* 107-117.

Jones, E. E., & Davis, K. E. (1965). From Acts to dispositions: The attribution process in person perception. In L. Berkowitz (Ed.), *Advances in Experimental Social Psychology* (Vol. 2), New York, Academic Press.

Konečni, V. J. (1979). The role of aversive events in the development of intergroup conflict. In W. G. Austin & S. Worchel (Eds.), *The social psychology of intergroup relations*. Monterey, CA: Brooks/Cole.

Kulik, J. A. (1983). Confirmatory attribution and the perpetuation of social beliefs. *Journal of Personality and Social Psychology, 44,* 1171-1181.

LeVine, R. A., & Campbell, D. T. (1972). *Ethnocentrism: Theories of conflict, ethnic attitudes and group behavior.* New York: Wiley.

Lewin, K. (1948). *Resolving social conflicts.* New York: Harper & Row.

Linville, P. W., & Jones, E. E. (1980). Polarized appraisals of outgroup members. *Journal of Personality and Social Psychology, 38,* 689-703.

Locksley, A., Borgida, E., Brekke, N., & Hepburn, C. (1980). Sex stereotypes and social judgement. *Journal of Personality and Social Psychology, 39,* 821-831.

Locksley, A., Hepburn, C., & Ortiz, V. (1982). Social stereotypes and judgments of individuals: An instance of the base rate fallacy. *Journal of Experimental Social Psychology, 18,* 23-42.

Mackie, J. L. (1974). *The cement of the universe: A study of causation.* Oxford: Clarendon.

Malpass, R. S., & Kravitz, J. (1969). Recognition for faces of own and other race. *Journal of Personality and Social Psychology, 13,* 330-334.

Manis, M. (1977). Cognitive social psychology. *Personality and Social Psychology Bulletin, 3,* 550-556.

Mazrui, A. A. (1980). *The African condition.* London: Heinemann.

McArthur, L. Z. (1982). Judging a book by its cover. A cognitive analysis of the relationship between physical appearance and stereotyping. In A. Hastorf & A. Isen (Eds.). *Cognitive social psychology.* New York: Elsevier North-Holland.

McArthur, L. Z., & Post, D. L. (1977). Figural emphasis and person perception. *Journal of Experimental Social Psychology, 13,* 520-535.

Merton, R. K. (1957). *Social theory and social structure.* Glencoe, IL: Free Press.

Michotte, A. E. (1946), *La perception de la causalité.* Paris: J. Vrin (In Translation, *The perception of causality.* New York: Basic Books, 1963).

Miller, D. T., & Ross, M. (1975). Self-serving biases in the attribution of causality: Fact or fiction?. *Psychological Bulletin, 82,* 213-225.

Myrdal, G. (1944). *An American dilemma.* New York: Harper.

Nisbett, R., & Ross, L. (1980). *Human inference: Strategies and shortcomings of social judgment.* Englewood Cliffs, NJ: Prentice-Hall.

Pettigrew, T. F. (1979). The ultimate attribution error: Extending Allport's cognitive analysis of prejudice. *Personality and Social Psychology Bulletin, 5,* 461-476.

Pettigrew, T. F. (1986). The intergroup contact hypothesis reconsidered. In M. Hewstone & R. J. Brown (Eds.). *Contact and conflict in intergroup encounters.* Oxford, Blackwell.

Plon, M. (1975). On the meaning of the notion of conflict and its study in social psychology. *European Journal of Social Psychology, 4,* 389-436.

Poliakov, L. (1980). *La causalité diabolique.* Paris: Calmann-Lévy.

Pryor, J. B., & Kriss, M. (1977). The cognitive dynamics of salience in the attribution process. *Journal of Personality and Social Psychology, 35,* 49-55.

Pyszczynski, T. A., & Greenberg, J. (1981). Role of disconfirmed expectancies in the instigation of attributional processing. *Journal of Personality and Social Psychology, 40,* 31-38.

Read, S. J. (1983). Once is enough. Causal reasoning from a single instance. *Journal of Personality and Social Psychology, 45,* 323-334.

Read, S. J. (1984). Analogical reasoning in social judgment: The importance of causal theories. *Journal of Personality and Social Psychology, 46,* 14-25.

Regan, D. T., Straus, E., & Fazio, R. (1974). Liking and the attribution process. *Journal of Experimental Social Psychology, 10,* 385-397.

Rose, T. L. (1981). Cognitive and dyadic processes in intergroup contact. In D. L. Hamilton (Ed.). *Cognitive processes in stereotyping and intergroup behavior,* Hillsdale, NJ: Erlbaum.

Rothbart, M. (1981). Memory processes and social beliefs. In D. L. Hamilton (Ed.), *Cognitive processes in stereotyping and intergroup behavior.* Hillsdale, NJ: Erlbaum.

Rotter, J. B. (1966). Generalized expectancies for internal versus external control of reinforcement. *Psychological Monographs, 80* (1, Whole No. 609).

Sartre, J.-P. (1954). *Réflexions sur la question juive.* Paris: Gallimard.

Schwarzwald, J., & Yinon, Y. (1977). Symmetrical and asymmetrical interethnic perception in Israel. *International Journal of Intercultural Relations, 1,* 40–47.

Shaklee, H., & Fischhoff, B. (1979). *Limited minds and multiple causes: Discounting in multi-causal attributions.* Unpublished manuscript, University of Iowa.

Shaver, G. (1981). Back to basics: On the role of theory in the attribution of causality. In J. H. Harvey, W. Ickes, & R. F. Kidd (Eds.). *New directions in attribution research* (Vol. 3). Hillsdale, NJ: Erlbaum.

Sherif, M. (1966). *Group conflict and co-operation: Their social psychology.* London: Routledge & Kegan Paul.

Sherif, M. (1979). Superordinate goals in the reduction of intergroup conflict: An experimental evaluation. In W. G. Austin & S. Worchel (Eds.), *The social psychology of intergroup relations,* Monterey, CA: Brooks/Cole. (Originally published in M. Schwebel (Ed.), *Behaviour, science, and human survival.* Palo Alto, CA: Science and Behaviour Books, 1965.)

Simmons, R. (1978). Blacks and high self-esteem: A puzzle. *Social Psychology, 41,* 54–57.

Smith, E. R., & Miller, F. D. (1979). Salience and the cognitive mediation of attribution. *Journal of Personality and Social Psychology, 37,* 2240–2252.

Smith, E. R., & Miller, F. D. (1983). Mediation among attributional inferences and comprehension processes: Initial findings and a general method. *Journal of Personality and Social Psychology, 44,* 492–505.

Snyder, M. (1981). On the self-perpetuating nature of social stereotypes. In D. L. Hamilton (Ed.), *Cognitive processes in stereotyping and intergroup behavior.* Hillsdale, NJ: Erlbaum.

Snyder, M. (1984). When belief creates reality. In L. Berkowitz (Ed.), *Advances in experimental social psychology* (Vol. 18). New York: Academic.

Snyder, M., & Swann, W. B. (1978). Behavioral confirmation in social interaction: From social perception to social reality. *Journal of Experimental Social Psychology, 14,* 148–162.

Snyder, M., Tanke, E. D., & Berscheid, E. (1977). Social perception and interpersonal behavior: On the self-fulfilling nature of social stereotypes. *Journal of Personality and Social Psychology, 35,* 656–666.

Srull, T. K. (1981). Person memory: Some tests of associative storage and retrieval models. *Journal of Experimental Psychology, 7,* 440–462.

Stephan, W. G., & Rosenfield, D. (1982). Racial and ethnic stereotyping. In A. G. Millar (Ed.). *In the eye of the beholder: Contemporary issues in stereotyping.* New York: Praeger.

Tajfel, H. (1969). Cognitive aspects of prejudice. *Journal of Social Issues, 25,* 79–97.

Tajfel, H. (Ed.) (1978). *Differentiation between social groups.* London: Academic.

Tajfel, H. (1981). Social stereotypes and social groups. In J. C. Turner & H. Giles (Eds.), *Intergroup behaviour.* Oxford: Blackwell.

Tajfel, H., & Turner, J. C. (1979). An integrative theory of intergroup conflict. In W. G. Austin & S. Worchel (Eds.), *The social psychology of intergroup relations.* Monterey, CA: Brooks/Cole.

Taylor, D. M., & Jaggi, V. (1974). Ethnocentrism and causal attribution in a South Indian context. *Journal of Cross-Cultural Psychology, 5,* 162–171.

Taylor, M. C., & Walsh, E. J. (1979). Explanations of black self-esteem: Some empirical tests. *Social Psychology Quarterly, 42,* 242–253.

Taylor, S. E. (1981). A categorization approach to stereotyping. In D. L. Hamilton (Ed.). *Cognitive processes in stereotyping and intergroup behavior.* Hillsdale, NJ: Erlbaum.

Taylor, S. E., & Fiske, S. T. (1978). Salience, attention and attribution: Top of the head phenomena. In L. Berkowitz (Ed.), *Advances in experimental social psychology* (Vol. 11). New York: Academic.

Taylor, S. E., Fiske, S. T., Etcoff, N., & Ruderman, A. (1978). The categorical and contextual bases of person memory and stereotyping. *Journal of Personality and Social Psychology, 36,* 778–793.

Tetlock, P.E., & Levi, A. (1982). Attribution bias: On the inconclusiveness of the cognition-motivation debate. *Journal of Experimental Social Psychology, 18,* 68–88.

Triandis, H.C. (1979). Commentary. In W.G.Austin & S.Worchel (Eds.), *The social psychology of intergroup relations.* Monterey, CA: Brooks/Cole.

Turner, J.C. (1981). The experimental social psychology of intergroup behaviour. In J.C.Turner & H.Giles (Eds.), *Intergroup behaviour.* Oxford: Blackwell.

Turner, J.C. (1982). Towards a cognitive redefinition of the social group. In H.Tajfel (Ed.). *Social identity and intergroup relations.* Cambridge/Paris: Cambridge University Press/Maison des Sciences de l'Homme.

Turner, J.C., & Brown, R.J. (1978). Social status, cognitive alternatives and intergroup relations. In H.Tajfel (Ed.), *Differentiation between social groups.* London: Academic.

Tversky, A., & Kahneman, D. (1974). Judgment under uncertainty: Heuristics and biases. *Science, 185,* 1124–1131.

Ugwuegbu, D.C. (1979). Racial and evidential factors in juror attribution of legal responsibility. *Journal of Experimental Social Psychology, 15,* 133–146.

Ward, C., & Hewstone, M. (1985). Ethnicity, language and intergroup relations in Malaysia and Singapore: A social psychological analysis. *Journal of Multilingual and Multicultural Development, 6,* 271–296.

Weary, G. (1979). Self-serving attributional biases: Perceptual or response distortions? *Journal of Personality and Social Psychology, 37,* 1418–1420.

Weary, G., Rich, M.C., Harvey, J.H., & Ickes, W. (1980). Heider's formulation of social perception and attributional processes: Toward further clarification. *Personality and Social Psychology Bulletin, 6,* 37–43.

Weber, R., & Crocker, J. (1983). Cognitive processes in the revision of stereotypic beliefs. *Journal of Personality and Social Psychology, 45,* 961–977.

Weiner, B. (1979). A theory of motivation for some classroom experiences. *Journal of Educational Psychology, 71,* 3–25.

Weiner, B. (1982). The emotional consequences of causal attributions. In M.Clark & S.T.Fiske (Eds.), *Affect and cognition: The 17th annual Carnegie symposium on cognition.* Hillsdale, NJ: Erlbaum.

Weiner, B. (1985a). An attributional theory of achievement motivation and emotion. *Psychological Review, 92,* 548–573.

Weiner, B. (1985b). „Spontaneous" causal thinking. *Psychological Bulletin, 97,* 74–84.

Weiner, B., Frieze, I.H., Kukla, A., Reed, I., Rest, S., & Rosenbaum, R.M. (1972). Perceiving the causes of success and failure. In E.E.Jones, D.E.Kanouse, H.H.Kelley, R.E.Nisbett, S.Valins, & B.Weiner (Eds.), *Attribution: Perceiving the causes of behavior.* Morristown, NJ: General Learning Press.

Weiner, B., & Kukla, A. (1970). An attributional analysis of achievement motivation. *Journal of Personality and Social Psychology, 15,* 1–20.

Weiner, B., Nierenberg, R., & Goldstein, M. (1976). Social learning (locus of control) versus attributional (causal stability) interpretations of expectancy of success. *Journal of Personality, 44,* 52–68.

Wells, G.L. (1982). Attribution and reconstructive memory. *Journal of Experimental Social Psychology, 18,* 447–463.

Wilder, D.A., & Cooper, W.E. (1981). Categorization into groups: Consequences for social perception and attribution. In J.H.Harvey, W.Ickes, & R.F.Kidd (Eds.), *New directions in attribution research* (Vol.3). Hillsdale, NJ: Erlbaum.

Williams, R.M. (1964). *Strangers next door: Ethnic relations in American communities.* Englewood Cliffs, NJ: Prentice-Hall.

Woll, S., & Yopp, H. (1978). The role of context and inference in the comprehension of social action. *Journal of Experimental Social Psychology, 14,* 351–362.

Wong, P.T., & Weiner, B. (1981). When people ask "why" questions and the heuristics of attributional search. *Journal of Personality and Social Psychology, 40,* 650–663.

Worchel, S., & Norvell, N. (1980). Effect of perceived environmental conditions during co-operation on intergroup attraction. *Journal of Personality and Social Psychology, 38,* 764–772.

Word, C.O., Zanna, M.P., & Cooper, J. (1974). The non-verbal mediation of self-fulfilling prophecies in interracial interaction. *Journal of Experimental Social Psychology, 10,* 109–120.

Yarkin, K.L., Town, J.P., & Wallston, B.S. (1982). Blacks and women must try harder. *Personality and Social Psychology Bulletin, 8,* 21–24.

Zadny, J., & Gerard, H.B. (1974). Attributed intentions and informational selectivity. *Journal of Experimental Social Psychology, 10,* 34–52.

Zillig, M. (1928). Einstellung und Aussage. *Zeitschrift für Psychologie, 106,* 58–106.

Zuckerman, M. (1979). Attribution of success and failure revisited, or: The motivational bias is alive and well in attribution theory. *Journal of Personality, 47,* 245–287.

Chapter 4

Conflict as a Cognitive Schema: Toward a Social Cognitive Analysis of Conflict and Conflict Termination

Yechiel Klar, Daniel Bar-Tal, and Arie W. Kruglanski

An essential element in the make-up of conflicts is the subjective *knowledge* the parties hold concerning their relation. Such knowledge determines, first, whether the situation is characterized as a conflict, and, second, how the conflict is reacted to, affectively and behaviorally. This chapter looks at intergroup and international conflicts from the perspective of a theory of lay epistemology (cf. Bar-Tal & Bar-Tal, in press; Kruglanski, 1980; Kruglanski & Ajzen, 1983; Kruglanski & Jaffe, 1986; Kruglanski & Klar, 1985) dealing with the process of knowledge acquisition. According to this perspective, conflict is viewed as a specific content of knowledge, or as a specific *cognitive schema*. The specific content of knowledge contained in a conflict schema refers to incompatibility of goals between parties. A conflict situation is said to occur when at least one of the parties subscribes to the conflict schema. Thus, the retention or modification of the conflict schema may determine whether conflict is maintained or resolved.

The chapter consists of two major sections. First, we discuss the particular contents of the conflict schema and outline the knowledge acquisition process whereby all schemata may form and/or change. Second, we consider the implications of the present epistemic analysis for the reduction of intergroup and international conflicts.

Conflict as a Cognitive Schema

Throughout the present paper the term "cognitive schema" is used broadly to denote a semantic network of associated meanings (or implications) emanating from a particular core belief. In the case of the conflict schema, this belief has to do with the incompatibility of the goals between the parties. Once incompatibility between own goal and goals of another side has been recognized by the individual or the group, the conflict schema will be activated and the situation will be regarded as an instance of conflict. If Libya's goal is to become the leader of the Arab world, and Egypt's goal is the same, then one infers that there is an incompatibility of goals between these two countries. In this case, a conflict schema would be activated. This analysis holds that without the core belief – concerning the goals' incompatibility – a situation might not be regarded as a conflict.

A somewhat different theoretical approach regards conflict as arising from the incompatibility between actions (Deutsch, 1973). However, incompatible actions may not necessarily be perceived as conflicting. For example, a hand raised against another might be viewed as an unintentional or playful gesture. In the same way, military movements towards one's frontier might simply be seen as a maneuver (as Israel perceived Egyptian military movements on the eve of the outbreak of the 1973 war). Thus, conflict is not a mere property of the situation, but rather an inference made on its basis. The arousal of the conflict schema mediates between the situation and its eventual characterization as a state of conflict.

This view, which regards conflict as a cognitive schema with a specific content, allows a parsimonious analysis, based on the knowledge that has grown out of the cognitive studies of schemata, since it assumes that all the schemata (including the conflict schema) are formed and modified via the same process. Three following points serve to characterize the schematic approach:

First, schemata, once formed, govern to a great extent the encoding, organization, and retrieval of information (cf. Fiske & Taylor, 1984; Minsky 1975; Neisser, 1976; Rumelhart & Ortony, 1977; Schank & Abelson, 1977). Thus, accordingly, once a situation is defined as a conflict, consistent evidence will be collected to support this schema.

Second, some beliefs serve as a basis for different implications and associations which vary from individual to individual and from group to group. In the present case, goal incompatibility may mean different things to different people. For example, some political leaders may regard conflict as a highly undesirable state of affairs. For them, a belief about goal incompatibility (hence, a conflict) between their state and another might lead to negative affects of frustration and misery. Other leaders might consider conflict an invigorating challenge. For those, a belief about international conflict in which their state takes part may arouse positive affects of stimulation and satisfaction. Furthermore, a (core) belief about goal incompatibility may have different action implications for different individuals (cf. Kruglanski & Klar, 1985). For some it may imply attempts at appeasement and conciliation, for others it may suggest the need to manifest militancy and aggression.

Third, schemata are subject to great variation in their *availability* and *accessibility*. Availability refers to the presence or otherwise of a certain schema in one's cognitive repertoire, whereas accessibility refers to the readiness with which a given schema can be utilized (see Higgins & Bargh, 1987). With regard to availability, Kelley and Stahelski (1970) showed that people who viewed themselves as competitors rather than cooperators tended to regard an unfamiliar laboratory game as a zero-sum type game. These people exhibited more competitive behavior than people who viewed themselves more as cooperators. This finding might be explained in terms of schematic availability: the zero-sum (incompatibility of goals) schema is more available to competitors and hence is more likely to appear in novel situations. Accessibility might be demonstrated by some of the classic work carried out on the arousal of aggression, such as Dollard and Miller's frustration-aggression hypothesis (e.g., Miller, 1941) and Berkowitz's work on aggression cueing (Berkowitz, 1962). In terms of the present schematic approach, an event which is incompatible with one's goal – or the frustrating event – might serve to prime the conflict schema. Once this schema has been brought to fore, it then becomes more accessible to a subsequent, though unrelated, event.

In this section, we have presented some of the implications of viewing conflict as a cognitive schema. Now we will consider the process whereby all knowledge or schemata (including conflict schema) are formed and modified, according to epistemic theory described below.

Formation and Change of Knowledge Structures

According to the theory of lay epistemology (cf. Kruglanski, 1980; Kruglanski & Ajzen, 1983; Kruglanski & Klar, 1985), all knowledge structures are formed in the course of a two-phase process in which hypotheses are generated and validated. The validation of hypotheses is assumed to be accomplished deductively. By this we do not mean to suggest that most lay persons are expert logicians. By now ample evidence suggests they are not (cf. Wason & Johnson-Laird, 1972). It seems, however, plausible to suggest that lay persons typically validate their notions from relevant evidence. Relevance, in turn, is assumed to refer to some kind of prior connection presumed to exist between the evidence and the hypothesis. The nature of this connection is such that one feels justified in accepting the hypothesis providing the evidence was affirmed. It is *as if* the individual formally deduced the hypothesis from the evidence based on a prior if-then linkage *subjectively believed* to connect the two (for a more extensive discussion see Kruglanski, in press).

The case in which a hypothesis is "deduced" from the evidence is usually covered by the common phrase that the hypothesis is *consistent* with the evidence. However, numerous alternative hypotheses can be consistent with (or "deduced" from) the same body of evidence. In other words, an individual might unwittingly subscribe to numerous "if-then" beliefs connecting the same evidence with different hypotheses. On becoming aware of more than one linkage, an individual might experience an inconsistency or logical contradiction of an A–not-A type. This, in turn, may undermine the individual's confidence in any of the alternative hypotheses. Insofar as those assert different states of affairs they could not possibly all be true.

An inconsistency between hypotheses is typically resolved via evidence which is not commonly deducible or diagnostic (cf. Kruglanski, 1980; Trope and Bassok, 1983) with which one of the competing hypotheses is consistent while the others are not. Thus, the use of diagnostic evidence makes possible a decision among rival alternative hypotheses.

A central postulate of the lay epistemic theory is that the process of hypothesis validation does not have a unique (or natural) point of termination. In principle, at least, it is always possible to come up with further and further hypotheses consistent with the same body of evidence. Thus, the fact that we have any knowledge at all, or confer the status of firm fact on any of our hypotheses, demands an explanation. Within the lay epistemic framework such explanation has to do with factors which inhibit or facilitate the process of hypothesis generation. These can be classified into two broad categories: cognitive and motivational variables.

Cognitive Factors

Cognitive variables affecting hypothesis generation have to do with the knower's stable and momentary *capacity* to come up with ideas in a given domain. This has to do with the aforementioned *availability* of ideas in a person's conceptual repertoire and with their *accessibility* at a given point in time. In sum, a person might generate alternative hypotheses on a given topic to the extent that their component constructs were accessible. Otherwise, the person might be unable to conceive that things could be other than they presently are, or to imagine "possible worlds" distinct from current "realities." In terms of the present theory this is referred to as epistemic "freezing." In this vein, Holsti's (1972) analysis of the events which led to the outbreak of the First World War is a good example of the effects of epistemic freezing due to cognitive factors. During the crucial and tense days following the Sarajevo assassination, the incapacity of various European heads of staff to generate alternative ideas to those that were so well thought out and rehearsed by themselves and their staff (i.e., the full mobilization of their armies) contributed to the outbreak of the war.

Motivational Factors

The lay epistemic analysis identifies three motivational factors affecting the hypothesis generation process. These are: the need for structure, the fear of invalidity, and need for conclusional contents. *The need for cognitive structure* is the desire to have clear and firm knowledge on a given topic; any knowledge as opposed to ambiguity, doubt, or confusion. This need might stem from various possible sources such as intolerance of ambiguity (cf. Frenkel-Brunswik, 1949; Smock, 1955), pressure of time, an obligation to reach a decision, or the need for immediate action. Arousal of the need for structure in a given domain may often dispose one to quickly generate a pertinent hypothesis and refrain from probing it too deeply or confronting it with further, potentially embarassing evidence or alternative explanations. This need might affect various seemingly unrelated phenomena which, at bottom, might all represent epistemic freezing. It reflects such phenomena as primacy effects in impression formation (cf. Asch, 1946; Luchins, 1957), ethnic stereotyping (cf. Hamilton, 1979), numerical anchoring (cf. Tversky & Kahneman, 1974) and belief perseverance (cf. Ross, Lepper, & Hubbard, 1975). For detailed discussion and empirical evidence relating the need for structure to the above phenomena see Kruglanski and Freund (1983), Freund, Kruglanski, and Schpitzajzen (1985), and Kruglanski (in press).

A heightened need for structure is thus assumed to promote the freezing of any hypothesis or schema, including the *conflict schema*. Labeling the situation as conflict provides a simple and clear-cut definition and dispels whatever ambiguity might have existed. Such definition allows for well-defined responses and removes the need for time-consuming informational search and deliberation. There exists by now much evidence from real and simulated international and intergroup conflicts that in confrontational situations, where indecision might prove dangerous, intolerance for ambiguity increases (e.g., Driver, 1962; Singer, 1958; Streufert & Fromkin, 1969; Suedfeld & Tetlock, 1977). According to the present analysis this should intensify the tendency to freeze on a clear-cut conflict schema, and to view the situation in simplest (e.g., zero-sum) possible terms.

It should also be noted that under high need for structure, reaching any clear structure represents a desired state of affairs. Thus, if such a need tends to be aroused during dangerous confrontations one would expect the emergence of additional simplistic structures, e.g., the perception of third parties as unqualifiably friendly, or of one's allies as thoroughly cooperative. Such hypotheses could be fruitfully pursued in subsequent research.

A second motivation assumed to affect the hypothesis generation process is the *fear of invalidity*. This particular concern stems from all kinds of anticipated costs of a mistaken judgment, e.g., costs to one's private or public esteem, to one's economic or physical welfare, to one's safety or freedom, etc. The arousal of fear of invalidity might facilitate a general unfreezing of the epistemic process. This might express itself in the generation of numerous alternative hypotheses and/or in increased attentiveness to relevant information.

Admittedly, the fear of invalidity might not be a predominant motivation of parties in conflict. They might often be more interested in upholding a particular self-serving view of the situation than in the grasping of truth per se (cf. Bar-Tal & Geva, 1985). One condition which might contribute to a more critical test of conflict-related beliefs is the parties' desire to be (or appear) moral and righteous. This might occur either to satisfy a demanding self-image, or to vindicate oneself in the eyes of a judging world, especially when its support and sympathy are badly needed.

Another condition under which fear of invalidity might be aroused is when one's confidence in previous beliefs has been shaken by overwhelming evidence to the contrary. Consider, for instance, Janis' (1972) analysis of transformation in the decision-making process of the Kennedy administration between the Bay of Pigs fiasco and the October Missile Crisis. According to Janis, the trauma of the former event shocked the administration into adopting a more careful approach to crisis management. Just as the fear of invalidity construct would imply, this led to the consideration of alternative scenarios, a closer examination of evidence inconsistent with the accepted views, and systematic playing of the role of devil's advocate.

A dramatic failure of existing policies may represent a case in which previously held beliefs are countered by salient contradictory evidence. In the absence of such evidence, however, a fear of invalidity might be induced by a contrary view held by a highly trusted "epistemic authority" (cf. Kruglanski & Jaffe, 1986). Indeed, it has been suggested (cf. Rubin, 1980; Wall, 1981) that much of the effectiveness of third party intervention (Fisher, 1983) might be ascribed to its capacity to function as such epistemic authority (cf. Bar-Tal & Geva, 1985). This capacity might derive from personal attributes such as wisdom or impartiality, as well as from the party's external resources (e.g., political power). Kissinger's Middle East shuttle missions between 1974 and 1975 exemplify the utilization by a third party of a wide array of resources.

While heigthened fear of invalidity might often inspire a renewed examination of conflict-related beliefs, it does not guarantee that such beliefs will be modified. Occasionally, closer inspection will only serve to reveal how "real" and deeply-rooted the conflict actually is. This has been noted by the sociologists of conflict (e.g., Dahrendorf, 1959) as well as by social psychologists studying the contact hypothesis of conflict reduction (cf. Ben Ari & Amir, this volume).

While heightened need for cognitive structure is assumed usually to effect a freezing of existing beliefs (e.g., comprising a given conflict schema), and fear of invalidity an unfreezing of such beliefs, a third motivational category, that of *conclusional needs,* is assumed to effect either freezing or unfreezing depending on the degree to which a given belief is congruent with the individual's wishes and desires. A conclusional need is the need to uphold a conclusion of a particular content. In fact, almost any conclusion could appear desirable to some person in some circumstances, for example, the conclusion that one is morally right, that one's adversary's claims are unfounded, or that one is invincible and impervious to attack.

The preference for specific conclusions may dispose a person to generate alternatives to an undesirable belief, or to refrain from generating alternatives to a desirable belief. As already noted, the first case depicts the process of unfreezing, and the second one of freezing. Sometimes a conclusional need might induce a preference for ambiguity, if the only unambiguous information available seems painful and unpleasant (cf. Snyder & Wicklund, 1981). At other times, such need might lead to bolstering of one's preferred alternative (cf. Beckmann & Kuhl, 1984).

A handful of specific wishes and fears may serve to reinforce and maintain (i.e., freeze) conflict schemata in the context of numerous intergroup and international relations. One such wish might be to preserve the preferred ideology, image of self and other and of reality. In this vein, Finlay, Holsti, & Fagen (1967) traced a large part of the policies of former American Secretary of State, John Foster Dulles, to his puritan ideology and commitment to Christian ethics. This induced a strong aversion to Soviet communism which, according to Dulles, rejected Christian principles, promoted atheism, and preached a new social order.

Somewhat similarly, personal ideologies either cooperative or competitive have been found to affect behavior in social psychological studies of dyadic interactions (Eiser & Tajfel, 1972; Kelley & Stahelski, 1970). The wish to preserve one's pride or "save face" has also been noted to induce avoidance of compromise strategies in laboratory studies of gaming behavior as well as in real-life international conflicts (see, e.g., Bar-Tal, 1984; Kaplowitz, 1976, for discussion of this particular factor in the context of the Middle East conflict).

A conclusional need occasionally contributing to the freezing of an international conflict schema is rooted in the fear of a surprise attack (cf. Bar-Tal, 1984). This may typically involve two separate components, distrust of the other's intentions, and distrust of one's own ability to thwart possible aggression. This leads to the perception of the other party as having malevolent intentions and a rejection of possible benign interpretations of its actions. Such patterns are readily recognizable in several longstanding international conflicts. Thus, Bronfenbrenner (1964) has suggested that many Russian beliefs about the West can be understood in the perspective of their fears of a Western attack. Similarly, Gamson (1968) analyzed three American positions with regard to Soviet intentions in the Cold War and concluded that assumed level of threat is a major determinant of remaining beliefs related to the American-Soviet conflict. Several studies (e.g., Heradstveit, 1981; Mroz, 1980) have revealed parallel perceptions of threat among Arab and Israeli respondents.

The aforementioned needs may represent specific cases of conclusional needs, which indicate a biased motivational influence on cognitions swaying them toward *contents* of desirable judgments and beliefs. Occasionally, however, the preferential feature of given conclusions might relate to aspects other than their contents, for instance to their novelty. According to this need, people may become bored of ideas which they have held for a long time, in the same sense that they grow weary of old clothes and discard them. Thus, on some occasions, a new idea might be adopted simply on the basis of its being different from old ones (even irrespective of its validity). Under this need, people might grow weary of a given conflict schema and welcome an opportunity to exchange it for an alternative, new conception. Sadat's dramatic visit to Jerusalem in 1977, following decades of bitter strife between Egypt and Israel, represents an instance in which attractiveness of an "off-beat" idea might have facilitated the reduction of a firmly entrenched conflict. It is well to remember that Sadat's conception was utterly different from conventional notions about reducing the Egyptian-Israeli conflict in a piecemeal, gradual fashion through mutual concessions.

Conflict Termination

Our epistemic approach assumes that the termination of a conflict is dependent on cognitive change – the unfreezing of the cognitive schema, or simply its relegation into a less central position in the cognitive system – by the individuals or groups that are involved in it. Conversely, the maintenance and the enhancement of conflicts are dependent upon the freezing of the conflict schema, or by its centralization.

This strictly cognitive analysis of conflict may look somewhat strange at first glance. Conflicts, as we all know, do not occur solely on a cognitive level; they are accompanied by acts. We realize that conflicts usually end due to one party being defeated by an adversary, or because one side has abandoned the field, or because the two parties reached a compromise. However, we suggest that any of these acts must be accompanied by the complementary cognitive unfreezing of the conflict schema, or by its relegation to obscurity, in order for a conflict to be in fact terminated. Failure to do so results in maintenance of the conflict situation. This can be illustrated by the anecdote of the loyal Japanese soldiers who continued to fight the Second World War twenty years after its end, simply because "nobody bothered to tell them it was over."

We shall try to avoid here a debate, of the "chicken or egg" style, concerning what comes first – the cognitive change or behavioral acts that reflect the cessation of the conflict. Evidence exists for both kinds of conflict termination sequences. In any event, cognitive change seems to be a necessary element of any conflict settlement. Cognitive change can be achieved through two distinct modes. The first mode is viewed as *conflict resolution,* while the latter is referred to as *conflict dissolution.*

Conflict Resolution

In trying to resolve a conflict, the conflict schema is attacked head on. This might be accomplished by rendering accessible evidence inconsistent with the schema's content and/or by arousing epistemic motivations working to "unfreeze" the conflict schema. Based on the core contents of the conflict schema, its undermining might require one of three types of evidence: (a) that one is not really striving to attain the goal believed incompatible with the other party's; (b) that the other party is not actually striving to achieve its assumed goal; (c) that the two goals are not actually incompatible.

Elimination of one's own goal (incompatible with another's) might be accomplished in any number of ways. A goal may be abandoned because it no longer appears attractive, because it is believed to have been attained, or, conversely, because it appears unattainable and therefore likely to engender only frustration and pain. An example of the elimination of a goal is recognizable in the change in American policy between the Carter and the first Reagan administration. A great number of conflicts experienced in United States foreign policy during the Carter administration originated from the goal of preserving human rights, especially in South America. When this goal was abandoned with the onset of the Reagan era, many international sources of conflict in which the United States was embroiled simply vanished.

An interesting form of goal change is goal partition, where a major goal is separated into a more attainable group of subgoals. Fisher (1969), who has advocated this mode of conflict resolution, cites several instances in which it appears to have led to an abatement of conflict. For example, an air rights agreement was struck between the United States and the Soviet Union during the Cold War because of a decision to exclude this issue from the broad concerns on which the major powers were divided.

Not every goal change by one of the conflicted parties automatically results in conflict termination. Sometimes, the other party might pose new unacceptable demands, or shift its goals in conflict, which results in an enhancement rather than in a reduction of a conflict. Iraq, which started the Persian Gulf War with Iran, has abandoned its original goal of conquering Iranian land. Meantime, however, Iran has set itself new goals incompatible with Iraq's, notably to replace the Iraqi President and to receive war compensation. This may have considerably prolonged the conflict between these two nations. Another case in which goal change by one party did not contribute to the reduction of conflict is exemplified in the concessions that the Polish regime made to the Solidarity movement, which served to prompt additional, conflicting demands.

Conflict may also be resolved through a change in the perception of the goals of the other party. This is attainable through various means, such as by believing that the other party has abandoned its incompatible goals, or by realizing that it did not hold them from the beginning. This may have been exemplified in the gradual change in Japanese perceptions of the West during the latter portion of the nineteenth century. During that time, formal proclamations depicting Westerners as "beasts" and "barbarians" gave way to a different approach which valued the technological advancements of the foreigners and diminished the perception indicating conflicting relations with Western foreigners. The Japanese realized that the introduction of foreign elements into their closed society would not necessitate a cultural decline and also that the West did not necessarily intend to gobble up their country. After all, the European intruders helped the Japanese build their country into an economic and military power which they would later be forced to reckon with.

A further example of changing the assessment of the other party's goal is through changing the causal attribution of its deeds. From Kelley's (1979) discussion concerning "attributional conflicts," it appears that a conflict may be resolved by adopting a new attribution for the source of the other's incompatible behavior (See Hewstone, this volume). For instance, the attribution of a deed to a desire to harm may be replaced, for example, by a perception of the deed as a benign, unintentional act which is part of an unfamiliar foreign custom (such as with tribal war dances).

Another major route to conflict resolution is to bring about change in the assessment that the goals are, in fact, incompatible. One example of this way of conflict resolution is the Israeli-Egyptian Peace Treaty, signed when both sides were willing to believe that their goals can be concurrently achieved. Israel achieved security without occupying the Sinai peninsula and Egypt got its land back without striking against Israel. (See Fisher & Ury, 1981, for a similar analysis.)

Conflict Dissolution

While conflict resolution often entails active focusing on the conflict schema, leading to a reassessment of its validity, conflict dissolution may occur when the conflict schema shifts out of the focus of attention and moves into relative obscurity. Research by Higgins, Bargh, and Lombardi (1985) suggests that the recency as well as the frequency of priming a construct or a schema determines its subsequent accessibility. Thus, a conflict schema left "unprimed" for long stretches of time might become relatively inaccessible and thus cease to exert important influence on judgments and behavior. For instance, a married couple could at one time experience intense conflict and react to it by negative affect, derogatory cognitions, and possibly negative actions as well. At a different time, however, after the conflict schema has been let alone for a while, awareness of conflict might grow more obscure and the negative thoughts might be supplanted by more positive notions such as "love," or "partnership." If this occurs, the same couple that only recently was on the verge of breaking up could now exhibit authentic affection and mutual commitment.

The same principle may also apply to groups and group members. People from two opposing groups, say Israelis and Palestinians, may maintain relatively positive everyday contacts (e. g., in the domains of commerce or labor) until such time at which the Palestinian-Israeli conflict schema surfaces in a group member's phenomenology. When this occurs, the individual's attitudes can shift drastically, to the point of undertaking hostile and violent actions towards persons with regard to which, under different circumstances, (s)he might exhibit genuine humanity and affection. Similarly, two groups may at one time be in intense conflict, whereas at some subsequent time they may experience warm and friendly relations, even though no systematic resolution of the conflict has taken place. The relations between China and the United States or France and West Germany may represent cases in point.

Decentralization of the conflict schema may take place as a result of changing conditions. Thus, the retrieval cues for the schema might diminish in saliency. Alternatively, other schemata may come to the forefront of people's attention, instead of the conflict-related beliefs. For example, the appearance of a superordinate goal common to hitherto conflicting groups may reduce the awareness of conflict. Thus, in the classic research by Sherif, Harvey, White, Hood, and Sherif (1961), conflict between two competing groups of boys was reduced via the introduction of a series of different superordinate goals which they shared in common. However, a decline in the accessibility of a given conflict schema may be temporary rather than permanent. For example, the United States and the USSR put their disagreements aside during the Second World War in order to cooperate against a common enemy; however, immediately following the victory over Nazi Germany, the two powers reverted to their conflicted relations, which have persisted ever since.

Summary and Conclusions

International and intergroup conflicts have been presently viewed in terms of the notion of "conflict schema", denoting a belief in the incompatibility of goals held by the parties. It has been noted that beyond the experienced conflict, schemata held by different persons (and/or by the same persons at different times) may vary considerably in terms of their affective and behavioral implications. Once a conflict schema is accessed and focalized in an individual's awareness it is likely to affect his or her affective experiences and conduct in the conflict situation.

The present approach suggests two modes of conflict termination: (a) *conflict resolution,* whereby the conflict schema is "unfrozen" via induction of the appropriate epistemic motivations, and confrontation with various types of inconsistent information; and (b) *conflict dissolution,* whereby the conflict schema, by being "left alone" becomes relatively inaccessible, thus ceasing to affect the individual's experience and behavior.

The present analysis does not intend to replace alternative approaches to conflict and conflict resolution. It adds a perspective which interprets conflict processes from the standpoint of a general social cognitive or epistemic theory. Furthermore, the proposed approach provides a framework in which previous works on conflict receive new meaning. For example, many of the previous contributions focus on specific modes of unfreezing and/or decentralization of the conflict schema (e. g., Kelley, 1979; Kelman, 1982; Sherif et al. 1961).

Such a framework may open new avenues for the study of conflict, stressing in particular the various cognitive and motivational factors affecting the unfreezing and refreezing of schemata as well as the processes whereby accessibility shifts may be effected. Hopefully, the approach proposed herein may yield practical as well as conceptual and empirical implications for our ability to understand and manage a variety of conflicts.

References

Asch, S.E. (1946). Forming impressions of personality. *Journal of Abnormal and Social Psychology, 41,* 88–92.

Bar-Tal, D. (1984). Israeli-Palestinian conflict: A cognitive analysis. Unpublished manuscript, Tel-Aviv University.

Bar-Tal, D., & Bar-Tal, Y. (in press). New perspective of social psychology. In D. Bar-Tal & A. Kruglanski (Eds.), *The social psychology of knowledge.* Cambridge: Cambridge University Press.

Bar-Tal, D., & Geva, N. (1985). A cognitive basis of international conflict. In W.G. Austin & S. Worchel (Eds.), *The social psychology of intergroup relations* (2nd ed.). Chicago: Nelson-Hall.

Beckmann, J. & Kuhl, J. (1984). Altering information to gain action control: Functional aspects of human information processing in decision making. *Journal of Research in Personality, 18,* 224–237.

Berkowitz, L. (1962). *Aggression: A social psychological analysis.* New York: McGraw-Hill.

Berkowitz, L., & LePage, A. (1967). Weapons as aggression-eliciting stimuli. *Journal of Personality and Social Psychology, 7,* 202–207.

Bronfenbrenner, J. (1964). Allowing for Soviet perceptions. In R. Fisher (Ed.), *International conflict and behavioral science*. New York: Basic Books.

Dahrendorf, R. (1959). *Class and class conflicts in industrial society*. Stanford, CA: Stanford University Press.

Deutsch, M. (1973). *The resolution of conflict: Constructive and destructive processes*. New Haven: Yale University Press.

Driver, M. J. (1962). *Conceptual structure and group processes in an international simulation: Part 1. The perception of simulated nations* (ONR Technical report No. 9). Princeton: Princeton University and Educational Testing Service.

Eiser, J. R., & Tajfel, H. (1972). Acquisition of information in dyadic interaction. *Journal of Personality and Social Psychology, 23,* 340–345.

Finlay, D. J., Holsti, O. R., & Fagen, R. R. (1967). *Enemies in politics*. Chicago: Rand McNally.

Fisher, R. (1969). *International conflict for beginners*. New York: Harper & Row.

Fisher, R., & Ury, W. (1981). *Getting to yes: Negotiating agreement without giving in*. Boston: Houghton Mifflin.

Fisher, R. J. (1983). Third party consultation as a method of intergroup conflict resolution: A review of studies. *Journal of Conflict Resolution, 27,* 301–334.

Fiske, S. T., & Taylor, S. E. (1984). *Social cognition*. Reading, MA: Addison-Wesley.

Frenkel-Brunswick, E. (1949). Intolerance of ambiguity as emotional and perceptual personality disposition. *Journal of Personality, 18,* 103–143.

Freund, T., Kruglanski, A. W., & Schpitzajzen, A. (1985). The freezing and unfreezing of impressional primacy: Effects of the need for structure and the fear of invalidity. *Personality and Social Psychology Bulletin, 11,* 479–487.

Gamson, W. A. (1968). *Power and discontent*. Homewood, IL: Dorsey.

Hamilton, D. L. (1979). A cognitive-attributional analysis of stereotyping. In L. Berkowitz (Ed.), *Advances in experimental social psychology* (Vol. 12). New York: Academic.

Heradstveit, D. (1981). *The Arab-Israeli conflict* (2nd ed.). Oslo: Universitetsforlaget.

Higgins, E. T., & Bargh, J. A. (1987). Social cognition and social perception. *Annual Review of Psychology*.

Higgins, E. T., Bargh, J. A., & Lombardi, W. (1985). The nature of priming effects on categorization. *Journal of Experimental Psychology: Learning, Memory and Cognition, 11,* 59–69.

Holsti, O. R. (1972). *Crisis, escalation, war*. Montreal: McGill Queen's University Press.

Janis, I. L. (1972). *Victims of groupthink*. Boston: Houghton Mifflin.

Kaplowitz, N. (1976). Psychopolitical dimensions of the Middle East conflict. *Journal of Conflict Resolution, 20,* 279–317.

Kelley, H. H. (1979). *Personal Relationships. Their Structure and Process*. Hillsdale, NJ: Erlbaum.

Kelley, H. H., & Stahelski, A. J. (1970). Social interaction basis of cooperators' and competitors' beliefs about others. *Journal of Personality and Social Psychology, 16,* 66–91.

Kelman, H. C. (1982). Creating the conditions for Israeli-Palestinian negotiations. *Journal of Conflict Resolution, 26,* 39–75.

Kruglanski, A. W. (1980). Lay epistemologic-process and contents. *Psychological Review, 87,* 70–87.

Kruglanski, A. W. (in press). *Basic processes in social cognition: A theory of lay epistemology,* New York: Plenum.

Kruglanski, A. W., & Ajzen, I. (1983). Bias and error in human judgment. *European Journal of Social Psychology, 13,* 1–44.

Kruglanski, A. W., & Freund, T. (1983). The freezing and unfreezing of lay inferences: Effects on impressional primacy, ethnic stereotyping and numerical anchoring. *Journal of Experimental Social Psychology, 19,* 448–468.

Kruglanski, A. W., & Jaffe, Y. (1986). Lay epistemology: a theory for cognitive therapy. In L. Y. Abramson (Ed.), *An attributional perspective in clinical psychology*. New York: Guilford.

Kruglanski, A. W., & Klar, Y. (1985). Knowing what to do: On the epistemology of actions. In J. Kuhl & J. Beckmann (Eds.), *Action control: From cognition to behavior*. Berlin: Springer-Verlag.

Luchins, A. S. (1957). Experimental attempts to minimize the impact of first impressions. In

C. A. Hovland (Ed.), *The order of presentation in persuasion*. New Haven: Yale University Press.

Miller, N. E. (1941). The frustration-aggression hypothesis. *Psychological Review, 98,* 337–342.

Minsky, M. (1975). A framework for representing knowledge. In P. H. Winson (Ed.), *The psychology of computer vision*. New York: McGraw-Hill.

Mroz, J. E. (1980). *Beyond security: Private perceptions among Arabs and Israelis*. New York: Pergamon.

Neisser, V. (1976). *Cognition and reality*. San Francisco: Freeman.

Ross, L., Lepper, M. R., & Hubbard, M. (1975). Perseverance in self-perception and social perception: Biased attributional process in the debriefing paradigm. *Journal of Personality and Social Psychology, 32,* 880–892.

Rubin, J. Z. (Ed.) (1980). *Dynamics of third party intervention: Kissinger in the Middle East*. New York: Praeger.

Rumelhart, D. E., & Ortony, A. (1977). The representation of knowledge in memory. In R. C. Anderson, R. J. Spico, W. E., & Montague (Eds.), *Schooling and the acquisition of knowledge*. Hillsdale, NJ: Erlbaum.

Schank, R. C., & Abelson, R. P. (1977). *Scripts, plans, goals, and understanding*. Hillsdale, NJ: Erlbaum.

Sherif, M., Harvey, O. J., White, B. J., Hood, W. R., & Sherif, C. W. (1961). *Intergroup cooperation and competition: The Robbers' Cave experiment*. Norman, OK: University Book Exchange.

Singer, J. D. (1958). Threat perception and the armament-tension dilemma. *Journal of Conflict Resolution, 2,* 90–105.

Smock, D. C. (1955). The influence of psychological stress on the "intolerance of ambiguity". *Journal of Abnormal and Social Psychology, 50,* 177–182.

Snyder, M. L., & Wicklund, R. A. (1981). Attribute ambiguity. In J. H. Harvey, W. Ickes, & R. F. Kidd (Eds.), *New directions in attribution research* (Vol. 3). Hillsdale, NJ: Erlbaum.

Streufert, S., & Fromkin, H. (1969). *True conflict and complex decision making: The effect of the three party duel and military and economic behavior of decision making groups in complex environments* (ONP Technical Report No. 25). West Lafayette: Purdue University.

Suedfeld, P., & Tetlock, P. E. (1977). Integrative complexity of communications in international crises. *Journal of Conflict Resolution, 21,* 169–184.

Trope, Y., & Bassok, M. (1983). Information gathering strategies in hypothesis testing. *Journal of Experimental Social Psychology, 19,* 560–576.

Tversky, A., & Kahneman, D. (1974). Judgment under uncertainty: Heuristics and biases. *Science, 185,* 1124–1131.

Wall, J. A. (1981). Mediation: an analysis, review and proposed research. *Journal of Conflict Resolution, 25,* 157–180.

Wason, P. C., & Johnson-Laird, P. N. (1972). *Psychology of reasoning: Structure and content*. London: Batsford.

Part III

The Maintenance of Conflict

Chapter 5

Social Identity and Intergroup Conflict:
~~An Israeli View~~ *A theoretical mastubatory view.*

John E. Hofman

Level of Discourse

The analysis of group conflict requires a decision as to the level of discourse at which that analysis is most fittingly applied. On the face of it, groups are molar units, high level abstractions, and the kind of people best equipped to deal with such units are sociologists. That is why conflict theory has for the most part been their special preserve (Coser, 1967; Dahrenhof, 1961). Psychologists who, on the whole, feel more comfortable with relations at the intra/interpersonal level, have respected the boundaries. What they would prefer to show is that group conflict is "nothing but" an extrapolation from private events. More typically, they have ignored the problem, with some notable exceptions (e.g.) Sherif and Sherif, 1956).

In the past few years, a group of social psychologists around the late Henri Tajfel has taken pains to explicate the difference between two kinds of group relations, those best described as interpersonal and those that are "real" group relations. Turner (1982), for example, makes a distinction between an interaction-oriented "social cohesion" model and a "social identification" model, the latter built around role identity. He finds the social identification model well adapted to the reality of individuals acting as group members rather than as private persons. In his own words, "Research should focus less on the determinants of interpersonal attraction and more on ... similarity, common fate, proximity, shared threat, and other unit-forming factors ... which function as cognitive criteria" (p. 27).

Indeed, it makes little sense to discuss serious group conflict at the level of interpersonal attraction or aversion, despite utopian visions of a scene where enemy soldiers wander into no-man's-land to embrace over a pint of beer. Unfortunately, wars are neither started nor ended in the manner of a private quarrel. Nor, in general, are labor disputes: good personal relations between management and workers surely will not hurt, but what is most likely to bring the dispute to a happy conclusion has more to do with collective bargaining and interpersonal contracts than with feelings of human kindness.

More to the point of the present paper, the Jewish-Arab Community Center in the City of Haifa routinely arranges for extended meetings between groups of Jewish and Arab pupils. Its carefully planned programs stress personal let's-get-acquainted games, home hospitality and picnics. For the first few meetings everyone is all smiles. Then, almost inevitably, someone raises a political issue, and, as if a switch had been thrown, all revert to ingroup justification and outgroup condemnation. Jewish and Arab persons begin to perform as group members. What Turner (1982) calls Tajfel's law will prevail: "As category membership becomes salient, there will be a tendency to exaggerate the differences on criterial dimensions between individuals falling into distinct categories, and to minimize these differences within categories" (p. 28).

Social categorization is the foundation on which the social identification model is built. The chemistry that turns the enemy one aims at through the sight of a rifle into the prisoner to whom one hands a cigarette marks a sharp change in categorization. The decision as to whether a person is an enemy combatant or an enemy prisoner determines our conduct towards him. Here again, Tajfel and his colleagues have taken the lead by demonstrating, in a series of imaginative laboratory studies, that the tendency of individuals to cluster into groups is so basic that it can be shown under laboratory conditions (Tajfel, 1970). Once group boundaries are drawn, social identity takes over. The question that hovers over every new encounter is, Is he/she one of "us" or one of "them"?

Social identity

Definitions

In a theory of group behavior the notion of social identity is most useful because it describes individuals in terms of multiple and hierarchical affiliations. People have as many loyalties as they have group identifications. Usually, though not always, they manage to avoid conflicting loyalties by shifting the hierarchy of their preferences from one social situation to another. This, however, is not always easy, as in the case of, say, Jewish Americans who feel strongly about their Americanism, but who also support the State of Israel. All they can do is hope that their attitude towards the Jewish state will remain consistent with United States policy. Thanks to an almost unlimited capacity for rationalization, most humans cope rather well with this and similar kinds on conflict.

Tajfel (1981) defines social identity "as that part of individuals' self concept which derives from knowledge of their membership in a social group (or groups) together with the value and emotional significance attached to that membership" (p. 255). The speed with which social identity can be engendered, once the basic categorization has been made, is truly remarkable. Nothing demonstrates the process so well, with respect to national identity, as the formation of new nations in the Third World. What only yesterday was a vaguely delimited colonial territory, inhabited by loosely bound tribes, almost overnight turns into a nation-state with a new name, a new flag, a new anthem: in sum, a new identity.

Still, one wonders, is there no difference between the kind of identity that arises, Venus-like, from the foam of this morning's events and the kind that has been molded over the centuries by common fate and adversity? No difference between being, say, a Zimbabwean, when just a few years ago, "Zimbabwe" was no more than a ruin in some remote corner of Southern Africa, and being the member of one of the country's historic tribes? The internal warfare that followed the establishment of the country suggests that there indeed is such a difference. The Israeli work on social identity, possibly because it focused on peoples with an ancient recorded history, has differed from Tajfel's approach in that it began with a historically grounded identity as its point of departure, taking categorization for granted.

In the 1970s Herman (1970, 1977), a one-time associate of Kurt Lewin, initiated a series of inquiries into the status of Jewish identity when that identity seemed to be submerged by the upstart Israeli one. The title of his 1970 volume, *Israelis and Jews – The Continuity of an Identity,* reflects concern over *lack* of continuity. Identity, he writes, "implies a relationship to the group beyond a given moment in time" (1970, p.22). There is something of a contradiction in Herman's reliance on Lewinian field theory, for it was Lewin who so heavily emphasized the ahistorical contemporaneity of social causation (1935, p.29). It was also Lewin, however, who wrote touchingly about bringing up the Jewish child so as to preserve the continuity of Jewish identity (1948, chap.11).

American theorists, true to an individualistic tradition have thought of the identity in interpersonal rather than intergroup terms. Rosenberg (1977), for one, has described "contextually dissonant" situations in schools, where individuals having a particular social identity (e.g., gender, ethnic, racial, or class) at variance with that of the majority, tend to suffer a decrement in self-esteem. Presumably, there would be no adverse consequences of that kind in a contextually "consonant" situation, such as an all-black or all-female or all-poor classroom.

When examining Israeli data on the self-esteem of young Arabs, however, it was found that a contextually consonant situation, the usual one in Arab schools, was no better than a dissonant one might have been (Hofman, Beit-Hallahmi, & Hertz-Lazarowitz, 1982). Apparently, in a heavily conflicted environment such as the Israeli one, context means something wider than the classroom. Adolescent Arabs think of themselves as Palestinians and as such compare themselves to Jewish youth, not to their classmates. Similar findings have been reported for black South African youth (Danziger, 1963).

In all fairness, Rosenberg (1979) does take this contingency into account and states that his generalizations "will not necessarily apply to all conditions that can appropriately be characterized as consonant or dissonant" (pp.125–126). How is one to resolve this issue of whether to regard social identity as the rapidly emerging product of categorization or as the luminous stage on which social encounters take their course? A balanced view suggests, perhaps, that one's *being* this, that, or the other minimally arises on a perceptual basis, but that a shared past surely adds to context, content, and rationale needed for in-depth evaluation.

Theoretical Basis

Following Lewin's (1951) field-theoretic formulations, and in agreement with later work (Herman, 1970; Hofman, 1970; McCall & Simmons, 1978; Rosenberg, 1979), one may regard identity as a dynamic configuration of traits, potentials, and behaviors as judged and labeled by self (ego identity) and others (public identity). Bridging the gap between the inner reaches of a person and that person's membership in groups, identity is Me on the way to becoming part of Us. As with Tajfel and his colleagues, social identity is viewed as a part of the total identity, or a "subsystem of the self concept" (Turner, 1982). Note, however, that Turner (1982) – as well as Tajfel (1978) – uses "self-concept" as the more inclusive term. This would seen to unduly restrict the subsystem of the self-concept to the realm of ego identity, leaving public identity out of the picture. In the present analysis, for the sake of consistency, "identity" or "personal identity" is preferred to "self-concept" as the more inclusive term.

A field-theoretic description of identity is like a map that stresses borders and regions, but leaves the exploration of the interior to the imagination of the research worker. This makes the approach somewhat abstract, which does not please those who wish to mine the rich ore of personal identity. In highlighting structural features, it has, however, the advantage of meeting the aim of field theorists to apply a unified system of constructs at different levels of discourse, in the interest of commensurability (Cartwright, 1959, p. 52). It also facilitates cross-cultural comparisons, as has been argued elsewhere (Hofman, 1985).

Miller (1963, p. 670ff.), whose lead is here followed, distinguishes between three concentric areas of identity: the ego-core, preserve of clinicians concerned with control and defense; a periphery. Jung's (1953) *"persona"* and Goffman's (1959) "presented self," the province of psychologists and sociologists studying person cognition; and an intermediate region, the band of sub-identities of special concern to social psychologists. It is this intermediate region in the main that is viewed as representing *social* identity.

The present approach is similar to Tajfel's in that it looks at identity as a force that relates individuals to their social environment, but it differs from it in several respects: for one, it deals with the issues that permit one to think of identity as a basic historical datum rather than as a lever for the enhancement of psychological distinctiveness; for another, it provides a rather detailed structural description that integrates the concerns of psychologists and sociologists; and, finally, it deals with multiple identifications that alternate in salience from one situation to another.

Subidentities

Of most direct concern to social identity and group conflict is the configuration of subidentities. These form specific links between the self and membership in groups. They differ in salience, valence, centrality, multiplexity, and interdependence, as well as some other dimensions of more specific interest.

Salience has to do with a subidentity's visibility in the field of subidentities. When an issue impinges on the individual's awareness, it "switches on," to use Turner's (1982, p. 21) phrase, the relevant subidentity by raising it to salience. It is not well understood why individuals become aware of an issue, considering the number of stimuli that compete for their attention, but surely a major factor in the social context is the extent to which they identify with the relevant group. Prolonged salience upgrades the subidentity in what McCall and Simmons (1978) call a "prominence hierarchy" and tends to enhance its *centrality,* that is, the importance it has among subidentities and the degree to which it is interconnected with them. *Valence* denotes the subidentity's attractiveness. It might seem at first that centrality and valence are practically identical concepts. While this is often the case, it need not be. When Lewin (1948), for example, described Jewish self-hatred, what he probably had in mind was an instance of a highly central ethnic subidentity associated with negative valence. Any part of one's being may indeed be very important, but not necessarily attractive.

Multiplexity has to do with the differentiation/integration of a person's subidentities. It would be of particular interest in a developmental study, but may also differentiate individuals operating at higher or lower levels of cognitive functioning. *Interdependence* characterizes the relation among any two subidentities, whether they are consonant, dissonant, or indifferent. To illustrate, the ethnic (Me as a Jew) and civic (Me as a citizen) subidentities of Jewish Israelis are positively valent and consonant, while they are dissonant to Arabs, given the difference in sign and centrality between being a Palestinian $(+)$ and being a citizen of the State $(-)$ (Hofman & Rouhana, 1976). According to Herman's interpretation of field theory (1970, p. 29), salience and valence interact to determine the subidentity's *potency,* that is, its ability to influence behavior.

With two further, closely associated dimensions, a *collective subidentity* and *solidarity,* one moves from the individual level to that of the group. The collective (sub)identity refers to awareness of and action on behalf of a commonly held subidentity. As Tajfel (1978, p. 39) puts it, "There will be some social situations which will force most individuals . . . to act in terms of their group membership . . . These situations, as they develop and continue, will enhance . . . the initially 'weak' forms of that group membership." Solidarity denotes a sense of common fate or interdependence (Herman, 1970, p. 208). It develops as the collective subidentity becomes more salient and valent (=potent) to group members, operates on „Tajfel's law" (Turner, 1982), viz., "intraclass similarities and interclass differences are enhanced as category membership becomes salient" (p. 28). Members of the „collective" will rally to the cause that pits them against members of the outgroup. In turn, group boundaries will go up.

As conflict continues, affect originating in the focal subidentity will spread to the ego-core, mobilizing defenses and threatening self esteem. „Any factors which cause or intensify group identification increase, by definition, the importance of that group for a member's self esteem" (Turner, 1978, p. 107). It is now Me and Us against Them, the original source of conflict hardly remembered. The Arab-Jewish conflict is not unique in having begun as a squabble over territory. What matters is that, in common with other such conflicts, it now involves and threatens the self-esteem of large numbers of people. This is all the more so as the national subidentity, which is the one at issue, would seem to be particularly volatile and likely to spill over to the ego-core. Arbitrated, goal-oriented solutions will no longer suffice. Collective egos, knee-deep in self-righteousness, will have to be diverted or transcended.

A description of social identity in terms of multiple foci has distinct advantages for an understanding of group conflict. In the main, individuals are willingly committed to such a conflict only to the extent that relevant subidentities are engaged. Thus, a work dispute may leave a teacher, doctor, or candlestick maker indifferent if the person is not involved *as* a teacher, doctor, or candlestick maker. Sometimes, commitment is situationally specific: on Friday evening, over cups of Turkish coffee, an Israeli Arab may feel strongly about the struggle for a Palestinian State, but by Sunday morning, on the job in a Jewish-owned factory, he could feel just as strongly about being an Israeli. What looks like inconsistency, or even insincerity, is a consequence of situational salience and multifaceted identity.

Measures of Identity

A theoretical conception can not be much better than the validity of its measures. The field of social identity has generated beautiful language, but crude operations. While some workers may regard this state of affairs as almost a virtue, others are at least partly committed to the ideals of quantification and operationalization. In our own work we have used a number of techniques to supplement extant ones, such as Kuhn and McPartland's (1954) "Who am I?" measure. In the next few sections, several instruments will be briefly introduced, namely, Likert-type questionnaires, the semantic differential technique, pair comparison, graphic representation, and open-ended questions.

Questionnaire

A Likert-type questionnaire can most directly embody the dimensions of social identity described in the previous section. The measures developed by Herman (1970) and his colleagues sought to operationalize validity, centrality, and so forth. They usually dealt with ethnic identity, but have been applied to other foci of identity as well (Hofman & Kremer, 1985). A typical questionnaire, dealing with the professional subidentity of teachers, is reproduced in the appendix to this chapter.

Semantic Differentiation

The technique developed by Osgood and others (e. q., Osgood, Suci, & Tannenbaum, 1957) has a special appeal, in that reliability is high and the purpose of assessment less transparent than in other techniques. Some evidence, for example, indicates that the hierarchy of prominence generated by semantic differentiation is more affectively tinged than one produced by the more obvious method of pair comparison (Herman, Hofman, & Peres, 1967).

Developing a semantic differential of social identity entails the systematic choice of a representative set of social labels (or concepts), including the self-concept (i. e., Me as I am), as well as of bipolar adjective scales able to differentiate the labels. "Semantic profiles" may easily be computed by summing and averaging adjective scale means over subjects. The profiles can then serve as points of departure for the computation of interconcept distances, really indices of the extent to which profiles differ from one another (Osgood, Ware, & Morris, 1961). It is an assumption of the semantic differential technique that *dis*similarity between profiles represents an estimate of the psychological distance between them. Conversely, similarity indicates affinity, mainly of an affective sort. The closeness of a label to the self, then, becomes a measure of identification. The more similar, for example, the profile of Israeli is to Me as I am, the more is the person or group held to identify with Israelis.

The intuitive validity of this procedure has been repeatedly demonstrated (Hofman, 1970, 1977; Hofman & Debbiny, 1970). When, for example, a set of labels includes Me as I am, Israeli Jew, Israeli Christian, and Israeli Moslem, the ethnic profiles of the three faiths will consistently be similar to the self-concept of Israeli Jews, Christians, and Moselms, respectively. In other words, Israeli Jews and Arabs will each "identify" with the labels denoting their ethnic identity. Obviously, labels may refer to any focus of social identity, thus enabling the researcher to investigate a large variety of social areas.

Graphic representation

In what may be called the "chessboard" method, subjects are asked to place tokens labeled to sample a conceptual domain onto a chessboard. The instructions are to arrange the tokens in such a way that distances among them express a subject's feelings about relations among them. The use of domain concepts and self-concepts yields data similar to those obtained by semantic differentiation, except that the direct and simultaneous manipulation of tokens makes the job much more transparent (Hofman & Mikhaelovicz, 1975).

An even simpler graphic method is to present subjects with bipolar continua marked by (it is hoped) contrasting concepts. Subjects check steps along *n*-point continua that correspond to their position. Some unpublished findings from Israel and pre-Zimbabwe Rhodesia indicate interesting differences between the two countries. In Israel, both secular and religious subjects felt strongly about being Israelis, as indicated by a preference of 3:1 for the Israeli side of the Israeli-private person continuum. In Rhodesia, by way of contrast, both Europeans and Africans favored the private person side to the Rhodesian one by similar margins. These 1974 data epitomize the difference in group loyalties in the two countries at the time, and anticipated the collapse of the State of Rhodesia.

Open-ended Questions

Open-ended questions, especially when used in conjunction with other, more structured measures, throw light on the meaning of statistical summations. A question such as "What does it mean to you to be X, Y, or Z," compensates somewhat for the loss in validity incurred by other instruments. Responses in this category can either be content-analyzed or reproduced verbatim for flavor, or both.

There is in none of the above a complete solution for the measurement problem in this "soft-minded" domain and much room for such more intensive methods as action research, psycho/sociodrama, and in-depth interviews, among others.

Application

The Israeli work on social identity, in applying the conceptualization of social identity outlined above, has been mainly descriptive and analytic (Farago, 1978; Herman, 1970, 1977; Herman, Hofman, & Peres, 1967; Hofman, 1970, 1974, 1977, 1978; Hofman & Beit-Hallahmi, 1977; Hofman & Debbiny, 1970; Zak, 1973). This has been useful in testing the versatility of the social identity model and its ability to make meaningful distinctions between individuals and groups professing various group loyalties.

When tension is known to exist between persons or groups, it becomes diagnostically useful to understand the extent of the commitment to conflict, whether it is relatively confined to the subidentity at issue, or whether it has spread through other areas of the identity system. A conflict is not always what it appears to be. For example, the internecine struggle among Lebanese groups has often been described as religious in character, that is, one between communities with long historical differences. According to some observers, however, the true nature of the struggle is actually socioeconomic and political. Whether either of these versions, both, or some others are correct is less important than the fact that a proper analysis of what is happening should take into account the differential involvement of multiple subidentities.

Description and analysis can also illuminate group issues in cross-cultural work. The gathering of equivalent data on the social identity of majority and minority members in the United States and Israel has furnished evidence concerning commonalities and discrepancies in two national settings (Hofman, 1985). Social identity theory and measurement high on structure and low on culture-specific content would seem to make certain cross-cultural phenomena more comparable.

Unfortunately, while description and analysis tell us much about what social identity is, they tell us too little about what it is *for*. Hence, it is important to study social identity in relation to its likely consequences. A beginning has been made in this direction, but the main work remains to be done. Social identity can be expected to bear on a great many behavioral outcomes. In the context of the present paper, conflict is the outcome of focal interest.

In one study, the hypothesis was tested that certain subidentities of Jews and Arabs in Israel are related to "readiness" for adequate social relations (Hofman, 1982). Results showed that the civic, vocational, and national subidenties are in fact related to social readiness, the first two positively, the last negatively. This has implications for ways and means to improve relations, provided of course there is interest in improvement. Another study indicated that the professional subidentity of teachers is an efficient variable in the prediction of the intrapersonal conflict known as burnout (Hofman & Kremer, 1985). There surely are many more situations where specific subidentities, or combinations thereof, can account for varieties of intrapersonal, interpersonal, and intergroup conflict.

Indeed, a case can be made for the contention that social identity is a theoretical position that can encompass conflict at its various levels. To the extent that different types of conflict can indeed be described in a common conceptual language, one gets a clearer picture of what different levels of conflict have in common, and also in what way they differ.

Intrapersonal conflict can often be translated into social identity terms by describing alternations in the salience, valence, centrality, and potency of overlapping subidentities at any one moment or over time. For a somewhat trivial illustration, one may think of a young person in "conflict" over going to a movie or to a party, assuming that he or she cannot do both. The two subidentities that are competing in this case are Me-as-a-movie-goer and Me-as-a-party-goer. The one that attains greater salience and more positive valence will have the potency to elicit the winning behavior. Intrapersonal conflict almost invitably involves the core area of identity, generating tensions and mobilizing defenses, and spreading from there to the identity as a whole (cf. Miller, 1963, p. 674).

In describing role conflict, Katz & Kahn (1978, p. 204) concentrate on discrepancies in role expectations, but devote a line or two to the conflict that arises when, say, a mother and housewife experiences difficulty in going out to work. This situation involves the continued interdependence of two subidentities, that of housewife and that of working woman. If the two have similar salience and valence, they will be in a state of almost constant dissonance, with possibly adverse consequences for the core area of the identity system.

Interpersonal conflict, rather than involving two or more subidentities within the same individual, will typically engage the same subidentity of two or more individuals. Here, too, core areas of the sparring partners will be invaded by affect, the self as a whole being viewed under attack. Two males having positively valent gender subidentities and contending, let us say, for the same woman would, in terms of the theory, experience a rise in the potency of their gender subidentity, some posturing of the presented self, and a threatened and aroused ego-core area.

Group conflict is different from either the intra- or interpersonal type in that it activates the *collective* subidentities. When it spills over to the core areas of many individuals, the cumulative effect can be devastating. This is because the emotion that accrues to the collective (sub)identity, with all its symbolic paraphernalia, is much greater than one would expect from the simple summation of affect over members. It is this generalized struggle of collective identities that makes some group conflicts so difficult to defuse and settle.

It has often been pointed out that conflict is not all bad. People mature partly by way of the struggles that go on within and between them. Groups form their collective identity through confrontation: labor movements grow out of strikes; interest groups jell into political parties; tribes become nations. Conflict raises barriers, compels poeple to compare themselves and their groups with others, and thus helps them achieve their social identity. The trouble is that, once achieved, the social identity keeps the conflict going. Conflict and social identity may well spin into a vicious circle.

To make the line of thought presented so far more cogent, a number of hypotheses will be proposed, in a somewhat speculative vein, to suggest a connection between social identity and its construkcts, on the one hand, and conflict behavior, on the other. While the main interest of this paper has been in group conflict, these hypotheses presume to cover conflict at its three most significant levels of discourse, the intrapersonal, interpersonal, and intergroup.

Hypotheses

1a. All types of conflict, intrapersonal, interpersonal, and group, are experienced as a rise in the salience of relevant subidentities, the polarization of valence, and the associated increase in potency.
1b. Prolonged salience of subidentities will deepen their centrality, thus widening interconnectedness with other areas of the identity system.
1c. Affect generated by the impact of events on awareness may invade the ego-core, threaten self-esteem, mobilize defenses and coping mechanisms, and spread to the identity system as a whole.

2a. Intrapersonal conflict, in particular, is experienced as either (a) incompatibility of valence and centrality, e.g., self-hatred; or (b) overlap of salient subidentities, e.g., approach/approach, avoidance/avoidance, and role conflict; or (c) fluctuations in valence, e.g., approach/avoidance conflict.
2b. Intrapersonal conflict will usually be associated with a spread of affect to the ego-core.
2c. Intrapersonal conflict need not affect the presented self.

3a. Interpersonal conflict, in particular, is experienced as a direct attack on the ego-core.

3 b. Interpersonal conflict will be associated with a spread of affect from the ego-core.
3 c. Interpersonal conflict will set social comparison processes in motion.

4 a. Group conflict, in particular, is experienced as an engagement of specific *collective* subidentities, generating solidarity.
4 b. Group conflict will be associated with a spread of affect to the ego-cores of group members.
4 c. Group conflict will set social comparison processes in motion.

What these hypotheses suggest is that conflict at any level is likely to spread to the identity system as a whole. Group conflict, due to the accumulation of affect, is particularly vulnerable to this development. When conflict becomes one between identities rather than over issues, the original cause of the conflict pales in importance. Arbitration by third parties no longer suffices. The threat to collective identities will have to be met by some method of diverting or redirecting collective emotion.

It may be of some interest to look at the work of Abelson (1959, p. 350) who describes four methods of conflict resolution, of which two, *differentiation* and *transcendance,* are particularly applicable. Differentiation, in the present context, means separatism, the physical disengagement of competing identities. Transcendance, in contrast, calls for the cultivation of an overarching social identity. Applying these formulae to the Israeli case suggests two widely advocated alternatives, either the establishment of independent Jewish and Palestinian states, or the integration of Jewish and Arab subidentities into a broad Israeli (or Palestinian?) supraidentity. The choice, then, is between separatism and integration. Great polities, like the Unites States and the USSR, have accomplished integration by way of pluralism and confederation. Smaller ones, like Albania or Israel, appear to prefer ethnic separatism. A closer scrutiny of political reality would show that some separatism occurs in the most integrated societies, and some integration in the most separatist ones. In the long run, a rational policy would seem to be one that attempts to tip the balance in favor of a civic supraidentity able to accommodate specific group loyalties as well.

Some Concluding Remarks

Social identity appears to be a promising conceptual framework for the clarification of group relations and conflict. This is so because social identity mediates between individuals and their world as members of groups. By this view, the group, rather than being merely a sociological abstraction, retains its existential status as a shared attitude among persons who have invested part of themselves in some social category.

Social identity has both structural and functional validity. Structurally, the comparison of prominence hierarchies throws light on the particular divergencies among individuals and groups. Functionally, the dependence of conflict behavior on identifiable elements in the identity structure suggests ways that may help individuals and group members isolate or transcend incompatabilities. The analysis of social identity may do no more than create awareness of conflict, pinpoint the issues, and help restructure perceptions, but, as a supplement to the initiation of social change, that is after all something.

Appendix

Questionnaire for the assessment of the professional subidentity of teachers

Please read the following statements with care and indicate by a circle around the appropriate number how you feel about each statement.

	Agree very much	Agree	Disagree	Disagree very much
It is important to me to be a teacher (C).	5	4	2	1
If I were to be born again, I would again choose to be a teacher (V).	5	4	2	1
I find it easy to introduce myself as a teacher (SP)	5	4	2	1
When a newspaper criticizes teachers, I feel as if I was were being criticized (S).	5	4	2	1
I feel joyful whenever I think of teaching (V).	5	4	2	1
In the teachers' room, I feel that I am among friends (S).	5	4	2	1
When people mistake me for anything but a teacher, I correct them (SP).	5	4	2	1
I like to think of teaching as a challenge (C).	5	4	2	1
I feel comfortable when the conversation turns to teaching (SP).	5	4	2	1
I am ready to join other teachers in fighting for better conditions (S).	5	4	2	1
The fact that I am a teacher has a great influence on my life (C).	5	4	2	1
I look forward to going to school in the morning (V).	5	4	2	1

Note: When respondent does not reply to an item, it is coded 3. C=centrality; V=validity; S=solidarity; SP=self presentation.

References

Abelson, R. P. (1959). Modes of resolution of belief dilemmas. *Journal of Conflict Resolution, 3*, 343–352.

Cartwright, D. (1959). Lewinian theory as a contemporary systematic framework. In S. Koch (Ed.), *Psychology: A study of a science.* (Vol. 2). New York: McGraw-Hill.

Coser, L. (1967). *Continuities in the study of social conflict.* New York: Free Press.

Dahrendorf, R. (1961). *Class and class conflicts in industrial societies.* London: Routledge & Kegan Paul.

Danziger, K. (1963). The psychological future of an oppressed group. *Social Forces, 62*, 31–40.

Farago, U. (1978). The ethnic identity of Russian students in Israel. *The Jewish Journal of Sociology, 20*, 115–127.

Goffman, E. (1959). *The presentation of self in everyday life.* New York: Doubleday.

Herman, S. N. (1970). *Israelis and Jews: The continuity of an identity.* New York: Random House.

Herman, S. N. (1977). *Jewish identity: A social psychological perspective.* Beverly Hills: Sage.

Herman, S. N., Hofman, J. E., & Peres, Y. (1967). *The identity and cultural values of high school students in Israel* (Cooperative Research Project OE-4-21-013). Jerusalem: The Hebrew University and US Office of Education, Health, and Welfare.

Hofman, J. E. (1970). The meaning of being a Jew in Israel: An analysis of ethnic identity. *Journal of Personality and Social Psychology, 15*, 196–202.

Hofman, J. E. (1974). Dimuyim leumiyim shel noar aravi b'Yisrael ubagada hamaaravit [National stereotypes of Arab youth in Israel and on the West Bank]. *Megamot, 20*, 316–324.

Hofman, J. E. (1977). Identity and intergroup perception in Israel. *International Journal of Intercultural Relations, 1*, 79–102.

Hofman, J. E. (1978). Tmurot b'haarachat dimuyim leumiyim-datiyim shel noar aravi b'Yisrael [Changes in national-religious stereotypes of Arab youth in Israel]. *Megamot, 24*, 277–282.

Hofman, J. E. (1982) Social identity and readiness for social relations between Jews and Arabs in Israel. *Human Relations, 35*, 724–741.

Hofman, J. E. (1985). Arabs and Jews, blacks and whites: Identity and group relations. *Journal of Multilingual and Multicultural Development, 6*, 217–237.

Hofman, J. E., & Beit-Hallahmi, B. (1977). The Palestinian identity and Israel's Arabs. *Peace Research, 9*, 13–22.

Hofman, J. E., Beit-Hallahmi, B., & Hertz-Lazarowitz, R. (1982) Self concept of Jewish and Arab adolescents in Israel. *Journal of Personality and Social Psychology, 43*, 786–792.

Hofman, J. E., Debbiny, S. (1970) Religious affiliation and ethnic identity. *Psychological Reports, 26*, 1014.

Hofman, J. E., & Kremer, L. (1985). Teachers' professional identity and burnout. *Research in Education, 34*, 89–95.

Hofman, J. E., Mikhaelovicz, R. (1975). Concept differentiation by semantic and visual differentiation. *Psychological Reports, 36*, 575–578.

Hofman, J. E. & Rouhana, N. (1976). Young Arabs in Israel: Some aspects of a conflicted social identity. *Journal of Social Psychology, 99*, 75–86.

Jung, C. G. (1953). *The development of personality.* New York: Pantheon.

Katz, D., & Kahn, R. L. (1978). *The social psychology of organizations* (2nd Ed). New York: Wiley.

Kuhn, M. H. & McPartland, T. S. (1954). An empirical investigation of self attitudes. *American Sociological Review, 19*, 68–76.

Lewin, K. (1935). *Dynamic theory of personality.* New York: McGraw-Hill.

Lewin, K. (1948). *Resolving social conflict.* New York: Harper.

Lewin, K. (1951). *Field theory in the social sciences.* New York: Harper.

McCall, G. J., & Simmons, G. J. (1978). *Identities and interactions* (rev. ed.). New York: Free Press.

Miller, D. R. (1963). The study of social relationships. Situation, identity and social interaction. In S. Koch (Ed.), *Psychology: A study of a science (Vol. 5).* New York: McGraw-Hill.

Osgood, C.E., Suci, G.J., & Tannenbaum, P.H. (1957). *The measurement of meaning*. Urbana, IL: University of Illinois Press.

Osgood, C.E., Ware, E.E., & Morris, C. (1961). Analysis of the connotative meanings of a variety of human values as experienced by American college students. *Journal of Abnormal and Social Psychology, 62*, 62-73.

Rosenberg, M. (1977). Contextual dissonance effects: Nature and causes. *Psychiatry, 40*, 205-217.

Rosenberg, M. (1979). *Conceiving the self*. New York: Basic Books.

Sherif, M., & Sherif, C.W. (1956). *An outline of social psychology*. New York: Harper.

Tajfel, H. (1970). Experiments in intergroup discrimination. *Scientific American, 223*, 96-102.

Tajfel, H. (1978). Interindividual behaviour and intergroup behaviour. In H. Tajfel (Ed.), *Differentiation between social groups*. London: Academic.

Tajfel, H. (1981). *Human groups and social categories: Studies in social psychology*. Cambridge: Cambridge University Press.

Turner, J.C. (1978). Social categorization and social discrimination in a minimal group paradigm. In H. Tajfel (Ed.), *Differentiation between social groups*. London: Academic.

Turner, J.C. (1982). Towards a cognitive redefinition of the social group. In H. Tajfel (Ed.), *Social identity and intergroup relations*. Cambridge: Cambridge University Press.

Zak, I. (1973). Dimensions of Jewish-American identity. *Psychological Reports, 33*, 891-900.

may I suggest to the author of this chapter that to sweep the streets has infinitely more value than this bullshit?

Chapter 6

Political Terrorism: A Social Psychological Perspective

Nehemia Friedland

Political terrorism is obviously not new. Politically motivated assassination, arson, kidnapping, and other forms of violence date back to the genesis of human society. However, in the last two decades the phenomenon has reached unprecedented and unforeseen dimensions. Terrorist groups proliferate (cf. Alexander & Gleason, 1981) and terrorist incidents now claim, on the average, more lives than ever before (Jenkins, 1983).

This chapter presents a social psychological perspective on political terrorism. It opens with a characterization of political terrorism, followed by an analysis of its causes, and closes with a brief consideration of reasons that have made terrorism a preferred mode of violent political action.

The Definition Problem: What Constitutes Terrorism?

The discourse on political terrorism is often clouded by definitional ambiguity and a lack of consensus as to what terrorism is (Bowyer Bell, 1978; Laqueur, 1976). Much of the ambiguity arguably stems from the tendency to use definitions of what is "terrorist" to label actors rather than acts. When defining the former, value judgment is almost inevitable. The aphorism, "one's terrorist is another's freedom fighter," underscores the difficulty of dissociating the pejorative labeling of persons and groups as "terrorist" from one's sympathy or opposition to the political ends they pursue.

The difficulty may be alleviated by drawing a distinction between the actors and the act. Criteria whereby a violent *act* may be labeled "terrorist" can be found, quite easily, by searching for commonalities among various definitions of terrorism. For example, Brian Jenkins (1975, p. 1) maintained that "the threat of violence, individual acts of violence, or a campaign of violence designed primarily to instill fear – to terrorize – may be called terrorism .... Terrorism is aimed at the people watching. Fear is the intended effect, not the by product of terrorism." Freedman (1983, p. 3) suggested: "Violence may result in death, injury or destruction of property, or deprivation of liberty. It becomes terror when the significant aim is not to attain these ends but, through these, to terrorize people other than those directly assaulted."

These definitions suggest, first, that terrorism is not the mere use of violence for political ends but rather its use as an instrument of intimidation; second, that terrorist acts are almost invariably aimed at affecting others than the direct victims. Thus, the bombing of a railway station in Bologna, Italy, or of a crowd celebrating the Munich Oktoberfest were typical terrorist acts. The killing of 83 in the first incident and of 13 in the second served no immediate purpose other than the sowing of fear among those who were not physically hurt by the explosions.

The minimal set of two criteria makes possible the distinction between terrorism and other forms of politically motivated violence. For example, the clashing of armies in war cannot be construed as terrorism, as each army primarily seeks to *physically* incapacitate the enemy. Fear, to the extent that it is aroused, is a by-product. By this argument, not all acts perpetrated by groups that are commonly referred to as "terrorist" are necessarily terrorist acts. Such a group may, for instance, rob a bank in order to gain needed funds rather than in order to intimidate. Lastly, consider the actions of oppressive regimes. Torture is the main method they employ (cf. De Swaan, 1977). Yet torture per se, abhorrent as it is, does not necessarily constitute terrorism. For example, torture is not a terrorist act when used to extract vital information from a prisoner. It turns into terrorism when employed to frighten into submission the population at large. Terrorist acts, then, are not the exclusive domain of groups that are customarily designated "terrorist." Nevertheless, the remainder of this chapter will refer to such groups, or, in other words, to insurgent terrorism practiced by nonstate groups. This is not to suggest that regime terrorism is insignificant. The focus on insurgent terrorism is only due to the availability of more data on this than on other types of terrorism.

The preceding characterization of terrorist acts indicates that terrorism is essentially a form of psychological warfare. Terrorist strategy, in other words, is not predicated on the maximization of physical damage and destruction but rather on the achievement of a potent psychological – emotional and attitudinal – impact on relevant masses of people ("Terrorists want a lot of people watching, and a lot of people listening and not a lot of people dead" [Jenkins, 1975, p. 15].)

As an illustration of this argument, consider the car-bomb attack on the United States Marine headquarters in Beirut on October 23, 1983, in which 241 American servicemen died. This incident subjected the United States administration to severe criticism by the public, politicians, and the news media, and was arguably a precipitating factor in the decision to evacuate American troops from Lebanon. Thus, a *single* terrorist incident profoundly affected a superpower's policy in a vital region.

The above example reveals an important facet of terrorist strategy and its sophistication as a form of psychological warfare. By inducing fear, political terrorists threaten the intricate relationship between the public and authorities.

More specifically, intimidation is used to turn the public into a pressure group, motivated by fear to compel authorities to give in to the terrorists' demands. Therefore, the successful application of political terrorism requires not only that fear be maximized: it must also be used in ways that discredit authorities, instill doubt in their competence and in the wisdom and legitimacy of their policies, and undermine public faith in the existing system of government. The essence of terrorist tactics, then, is the drawing of authorities into widely exposed confrontations and letting the public judge their course and outcomes. Terrorism is successful to the extent that it corners authorities in "no win" situations. Thus, for instance, when using hostage tactics, the sophisticated political terrorist might minimize rather than maximize ransom demands, such that authorities' refusal to concede would be perceived as unjustified intransigence while a concession, no matter how trivial, can be construed as capitulation.

In sum, political terrorism is not only a strategy of psychological warfare but also an indirect strategy. Its victory or defeat does not depend primarily on what the terrorists do but rather on the response they elicit from target publics and authorities (cf. Fromkin, 1975). As stated by Horst Mahler of the German Red Army Faction, "The strategy of the terrorist nuclei was aimed at provoking the overreaction of the state in the hope to stir the flames of hate against the state" (cited by Schmid, 1983, p. 185. See also Marighela, 1971).

The Roots of Terrorism: Applications of Social Psychology

References to terrorism are rare or practically nonexistent in the social psychology literature and a social psychological explanation of terrorism has yet to be developed. As a preliminary step, this chapter examines social psycholocigal theories and propositions as resources from which such an explanation might draw.

Attempts to explain terrorism in social psychological or any other terms can be hindered by the heterogeneity of the phenomenon. Terrorist groups range in size from a handful of active members to thousands. Their national composition is highly varied. According to one source, terrorist incidents in 1982 were perpetrated by members of no less than 75 different nations (US Department of State, 1983). Terrorists' stated motivations are diverse: nationalist, separatist, ideological. The ideological spectrum contains neo-Nazism and neo-Fascism, on the one hand, and Leninism, Maoism, Trotskyism, and anarchism, on the other hand. Some terrorist groups are religious (Catholic, Protestant, Jewish, Shi'ite Moslem, and Sunnite Moslem) while others have a racial motivation. To further complicate matters, many terrorist groups adhere to a composite social/ political ideology, with most present-day separatist groups having a leftist orientation. And there are some groups that are known to have replaced their original ideology with a radically different one (e.g., the Colombian M-19, which turned from right-wing populism to Marxism).

Despite the heterogeneity of terrorist groups and the diversity of their motivations, some generalizations are possible. First, terrorism is essentially a group phenomenon. Although the history of terrorism contains examples of loners who committed terrorist acts, most terrorist action is perpetrated by organized groups. Moreover, group processes are also evident in the targeting of terrorist activity. Schmid (1983) stressed this aspect in his definition of terrorism: "Terrorism is a method of combat in which random or symbolic victims serve as instrumental targets of violence. These instrumental victims share group or class characteristics which form the basis for their selection for victimization" (p. 111).

Second, political terrorism is an outgrowth of intergroup conflict. This generalization is perhaps too obvious to merit mentioning or elaboration. It is only presented in contrast to the view that terrorist behavior is a manifestation of personality disorders or psychopathologies (e.g., Kaplan, 1981; Mickolus, 1980; Morf, 1970; Stohl, 1983). Judging by presently available information, the assumption that terrorists are in some sense abnormal is questionable. In fact there is some evidence to the contrary. For instance, the famous Japanese terrorist Kozo Okamoto and members of the German Red Army Faction were examined by psychiatrists and declared to be completely sane and rational. In both cases no evidence was found for the existence of psychoses, neuroses, or unique personality makeups (cf. Crenshaw, 1981; Paine, 1975). This is not to deny the decisive role that individuals play in the dynamics of terrorism. However, as will be argued later, their influence must be examined as an element of group and intergroup processes.

Third, with the exception of regime terrorism, which this chapter does not address, terrorism is the "strategy of the weak." For instance, it is doubtful that the Palestine Liberation Organization would have waged against Israel a drawn-out terrorist campaign with uncertain chances of success, had it possessed the skills, manpower, and material to prevail in a direct, all-out war.

By setting political terrorism in the context of intergroup conflict, as a strategy employed by the weaker groups to effect social or political change, the above generalizations pose two questions that have to be answered in order to unearth its causes. First, what are the conditions that produce a movement for social or political change? Second, what are the causes or dynamics that turn such a movement to violence?

The Movement Toward Social or Political Change

Movements toward social or political change generally emerge in response to an actual or perceived, persistent denial of individual, social, political, or national rights. Hence, recent work on intergroup conflict, and particularly on the social psychology of minority groups, provides a rich source of possible answers to the first question posed above. Most useful among these is the proposition that groups will reject their minority status and the disadvantages it entails when at least one of the following conditions is met: first, the social system that imposes disadvantages on the minority group is perceived as *unstable;* second, the uneven distribution of power, rights, or resources within the social system is deemed *illegitimate* (cf. Brown & Ross, 1982; Tajfel, 1981; Turner & Brown, 1978).

This proposition appears to be entirely consistent with recent outbursts of terrorism. It may be argued that the evolution of democratic philosophies and social systems has fostered the view that a discriminatory stratification of society is neither unshakable nor legitimate. Moreover, the revolution in mass communication has helped disseminate, worldwide, the belief that social change is possible, as it has turned the success of some groups in improving their lot into models that other disadvantaged groups can hope to emulate (cf. Tajfel, 1981). Thus, if terrorism is viewed as a strategy of social/political change, its growing incidence may be explained as resulting from minority groups' increasing drive to claim and regain rights.

Although the preceding speculation is quite compelling, it cannot be accepted without some qualifications. That is, while certain cases of intense terrorist activity may be justifiably related to minority or other disadvantaged groups' growing assertiveness (Catholic terrorism in Ulster, Armenian and Palestinian terrorism), others cannot be easily explained in such terms. Salient examples of the latter case are groups that have engaged in domestic political or rather ideological terrorism, in countries such as West Germany, Italy, or Japan. Members of these groups do not belong to any identifiable disadvantaged minority. On the contrary, most of them are members of the privileged majority (see Russell, Bowman, & Miller, 1977), and they cannot convincingly justify their acts as a response to wrongs committed against them. Instead, they usually attribute their turning to terrorism to the suffering of others. For example, one of the founders of the German Red Army Faction, Horst Mahler, indicated that atrocities committed in Vietnam and the indifference of the German government elicited the terrorist reaction: "It was our moralism that led us to terrorism. Many of us (in any case Ulrike Meinhof and Gudrun Ensslin) came the same way. The German nation again was passive .... We had nothing to identify with [in] the West, so we identified with the Third World" (cited by Nagel, 1980, pp. 221–222).

It is clear that current knowledge on the social psychology of intergroup conflict and of minority groups cannot adequately explain the preceding examples. Aspirations for social change, expressed by the Baader-Meinhof group or by the Italian Red Brigades, cannot be viewed as a group's rejection of a minority status, and it is difficult to discern the social or political conflicts that turned such groups to terrorism. This difficulty has led some students of terrorism (e. g., Kielmansegg, 1978) to the conclusion that the attribution of terrorism to social conflict should be altogether rejected. Franco Ferracuti (1982) maintained that "available facts, at least in Europe, contradict [explanations based on adverse social conditions], unless they are seen as internal obstacles, not related to social realities .... Terrorism ... is fantasy war, real only in the mind of the terrorist" (pp. 136–137).

This rejection of the social antecedents of some terrorist movements is unwarranted. It largely stems from a distinction between conflicts of interest concerning the distribution of tangible resources, power, or rights, that are viewed as "real", and *ideological* conflicts that are "unreal," the figment of insane or irrational individuals' imagination. (Interestingly, the judgment that terrorists are in some sense abnormal is usually reserved for terrorists operating within the judges' own countries, and it is rarely applied to those operating in other countries.) Psychologically, this distinction is indefensible. For members of the German Red Army Faction or of the Italian Red Brigades, their ideological conflict with the majority or the establishment is as real as any conflict of interests.

In addition to reflecting a double standard, the rejection of social antecedents of certain cases of terrorist activity highlights possible shortcomings of conflict theories. These primarily refer to "objective" conflicts of interest between groups the boundaries of which are well demarcated. Hence the tendency to view radicals who are well-off members of the privileged majority and who cannot present personal grievances as waging a "fantasy war." A more reasonable alternative, however, would be the expansion of conflict theory, to include cases of *intra*group conflict whose core is ideological. Such an expansion will make the theory more useful for the explanation of the emergence of radical movements of social change.

The Turn to Violence

The drive to effect social or political change does not in and by itself explain groups' turning to violence. Groups aspiring to such change can act politically or, if such action fails, undertake nonviolent acts of civil disobedience. Therefore, to fully understand the emergence of political terrorism, the analysis of social change movements has to be supplemented with an analysis of group violence.

Social psychological explanations of group violence, civil strife, and rioting, as well as explanations offered by sociologists and political scientists, draw heavily on the frustration-aggression hypothesis (Dollard, Doob, Miller, Mowrer, & Sears, 1939). The adaptation of this hypothesis, which is essentially a proposition about individual violence, to groups was made by various authors in a straightforward fashion. Dollard et al., for example, attributed German anti-Semitism to the resentment that almost every German experienced after the treaty of Versailles and to the crisis in the economy a decade and a half later. Berkowitz (1972) placed the hypothesis at the center of his analysis of black rioting in the United States in the 1960s. Sociologists and political scientists (e.g., Davies, 1962; Feierabend & Feierabend, 1966; Feierabend, Feierabend, & Nesvold, 1973; Gurr, 1970; Lupsha, 1971) frequently employ the term "relative deprivation," which is conceptually close to the frustration-aggression hypothesis, to explain political violence. Among the latter, Gurr (1970) has contributed the most often cited proposition:

"Relative deprivations" (RD) is the term used ... to denote the tension that develops from the discrepancy between the "ought" and the "is" of collective value satisfaction, that disposes men to violence .... The frustration-aggression relationship provides the psychological dynamic for the proposed relationship between intensity of deprivation and the potential for collective violence. (p. 23)

Such direct adaptations of the frustration-aggression hypothesis are compelling in their simplicity (Van der Dennen, 1980). However, it cannot be taken for granted that a hypothesis about individuals' reactions applies directly to the behavior of collectives. Billig (1976) noted in his criticism of Dollard et al.'s explanation of German anti-Semitism: "This explanation is altogether too neat .... It is too fanciful to imagine that the Germans were kept in a state of increasing emotional arousal for fifteen years, and at the end millions happened to rid themselves of their tensions in an identical manner" (p. 150).

More generally, the theory of individual aggression does not explain the uniformity of group or mass behavior. The possibility that pent-up emotions in a group of individuals erupt simultaneously is a coincidence that is too difficult to contemplate.

Despite his criticism, Billig does not reject the frustration-aggression hypothesis as a key to the understanding of group violence. Instead he proposes a wider perspective that may bridge the gap between the individual and the group contexts. First, the group must "ideologise and articulate its discontent" (p. 156). In the absence of a unifying ideology that gives meaning to the discontent, individual frustrations and grievances will elicit disorganized individual action. Second, group violence, rioting, or rebellion must be examined as an intergroup process. For any group that acts to alter a political or social status quo there is almost invariably another group, typically the "majority," that strives to preserve it. Frustration drives not only the dissident group but also the majority, and threats on the privileges that the latter enjoys give rise to a "reverse" relative deprivation (Rosenbaum & Sederberg, 1974). Under such circumstances it is not always clear which group instigated the violence, but there is little doubt that violent action and counteraction perpetuate it. Moreover, the presence of a threatening outgroup enhances the unity and uniformity of each group's action which, as argued above, the frustration-aggression hypothesis cannot explain.

The preceding interpretation of group violence applies to some cases of terrorism. For example, the conflicts in Ulster and in the Middle East bred terrorism that can be linked to concrete frustrations and grievances. This interpretation appears less convincing, however, when applied to ideologically motivated, domestic terrorism, undertaken by relatively well-to-do individuals in Western democracies. For one thing, these individuals are not typical victims of adverse social conditions and it is therefore difficult to identify the frustrations and deprivations that motivate their turning to terrorist violence. Second, adverse social conditions that foster frustration and feelings of relative deprivation usually affect large groups. Yet, to date, only a handful have joined the ranks of such ideological terrorist groups. Thus, in order to maintain the frustration-aggression and relative deprivation hypotheses as grounds for a general explanation of groups' turning to terrorism, it is necessary to resolve two questions: first, what are the characteristics of the modern democratic state that frustrate privileged rather than disadvantaged segments of society? Second, why is it that so few undertake terrorism?

A tentative answer to the first question can be drawn from the sociological literature. Arendt (1983) proposed that the anonymity of the modern bureaucratic state fosters a sense of political helplessness and frustration that might lead some to terrorism. Bonanate, who wrote extensively about terrorism in Italy, regards the immobility and stability of the democratic state as the main culprit: "A society that knows terrorism is a *blocked society,* incapable of answering the citizens' requests for change, but nevertheless capable of preserving and reproducing itself" (1979, p. 197). In different terms, the discrepancy between individuals' desire to influence, to "stand out" and "leave a mark" on society, and their actual ability to do so constitutes a sufficiently potent frustrator to elicit violence.

This proposition has two important corollaries: first, the more stable and conservative the social and political systems, the wider the discrepancy between individuals' desire and ability to influence and, consequently, the deeper the frustration. Expressions that are consistent with this corollary can be found in justifications of violence that ideological radicals often present: "The fat, dumb, happy people wallow in their ignorance of the government's wrongdoing, and something must be done to wake them up" (Devine & Rafalko, 1982, p. 46).

Second, the more that individuals believe that they *deserve* to influence, the wider the discrepancy and the stronger the frustration they experience upon failing to do so (cf. Thibaut, Friedland, & Walker, 1974). This corollary provides one possible explanation for the baffling, significantly higher incidence of ideological terrorism in democracies than in dictatorships, as the democratic environment enhances individuals' perceived right to influence and thereby accentuates the discrepancy between their desire and their ability to exercise such influence. In addition, the corollary explains the involvement of affluent, well-educated, middle- and upper-class individuals in terrorism. It might be that such individuals perceive their social status as bestowing upon them the right or prerogative to influence. Hence, failure to influence is likely to be more frustrating to them than to lower-status persons.

Having identified a source of frustration that might drive well-to-do citizens of democratic states to terrorism, we are still left with the issue of numbers. As argued, immobility and blockades presumably affect many, but only a few become terrorists. This apparent inconsistency cannot be resolved without taking into consideration individual predispositions. That is, different individuals might react differently to failure to effect the social change they strive for. Some may become disillusioned and give up, some will persist in their quest for legal, democratic avenues of social reform, and only those that are predisposed to violence will adopt the terrorist response. It is suggested, in other words, that the emergence of terrorist groups is due to a convergence or interaction of social and individual factors. As argued by Crozier,

Men do not necessarily rebel merely because their conditions of life are intolerable: it takes a rebel to rebel. Look at it another way: some men or groups will tolerate more than others. If one describes conditions of life as intolerable, one begs the question: 'to whom?' (1960, p. 9).

Analyses of the process or sequence of events that led to the emergence of terrorist groups in Western Europe (e.g., Hess, 1981) support this interactive view. The origin, in most instances, was a widespread social protest movement. Confrontations, often violent, with authorities and failure to elicit a popular response led to disillusion and to the deterioration of the movement. Remnants of the movement formed small, clandestine groups which maintained little external contact and a fierce ingroup loyalty and cohesion. These circumstances enhanced the status of violent individuals within the groups, elevated them to leadership positions and allowed them to establish terrorism as the groups' preferred modus operandi.

Although an interactive explanation of terrorism appears reasonable, indeed obvious, it reveals little unless the relative importance of social and individual factors, or the "shape" of the interaction, is specified. I propose that individual predispositions to violence will have a relatively minor effect on a group's turning to terrorism under three conditions: (a) when deprivation is intense, the group is denied the satisfaction of basic needs and the exercise of elementary rights; (b) when the group has articulated and "ideologized" its discontent (see Billig, above); and (c) when group members have a strong group identity, the group is cohesive and clearly differentiated from the outgroup. Given these conditions, individuals' adoption of the terrorist response is not necessarily indicative of violent predispositions. Thus, for instance, it would be rather foolish to maintain that violent individual dispositions are the primary cause for the rise of the Palestine Liberation Organization. The predicament of the Palestinians in the wake of Israel's war of independence, the fact that many of them have since been refugees, and the emergence of a strong national identity and ideology provide a far better explanation.

Individual dispositions, particularly the disposition to violence, become paramount when (a) a radical movement does not aim to satisfy specific basic needs or to reclaim elementary rights but rather to implement a general social ideology; (b) this ideology is incoherent and unrealistic, and (c) the group lacks a unique, separate identity. Terrorist groups in Western Europe and North America exemplify this case. As already argued, the protest movements from which such groups sprouted were not composed of underprivileged, discriminated-against members of society. Their ideology was often incoherent (cf. Devine & Rafalko, 1982), and their group identity was arguably diffuse, as they were hardly distinguishable from the "majority" or the "establishment" against which they protested.

To empirically validate the proposed interaction it is necessary to show that members of, say, the Irish Republican Army or the Palestine Liberation Organization) are more heterogeneous in their predisposition to violence than members of the Italien Red Brigades or of the German Red Army Faction, and that the majority of the latter are strongly disposed to violence. Such evidence is extremely difficult to obtain, however, and at present the proposed interaction can only be indirectly supported with a consideration of the size of terrorist groups. It may be argued that groups which emerged due to political circumstances or necessity would attract a larger following than those which grew as an association of violent individuals. The data support this argument: while domestic, ideological terrorist groups in Europe and North America are composed of only scores of active members, groups such as the Palestine Liberation Organization have a roster of thousands.

Terrorism Versus Alternative Form of Political Violence

The preceding analysis specified conditions that turn groups to violence. It did not reveal, however, the reasons that bring groups to choose terrorist tactics over other known forms of violent political action. These reasons have to be identified in order to complete the inquiry into the causes of terrorism.

One possible reason has already been suggested by the generalization that terrorism is the "strategy of the weak." A successful, even spectacular, terrorist act can be carried out by a few persons, with limited experience and meager means. However, there are no grounds to suppose that this reason is more valid currently than in past eras. Therefore, this explanation is only partial as it does not adequately account for the unprecedented preference for terrorist tactics shown by dissident groups in recent years.

To provide a more complete explanation one has to shift the inquiry from *root causes* to *facilitating conditions*. That is, whatever the causes of terrorism might be, there is little doubt that social and technological development, particularly in democracies, have created ideal conditions for the practice of terrorism. For one thing, unrestricted travel and the ease of procuring weapons have reduced operational obstacles to a minimum. Secondly, a complex technological infrastructure makes modern states highly vulnerable to terrorist attacks and provides terrorists with easy targets. Third, and most important, the revolution in mass communication and the current capabilities and operating philosophy of the mass media dramatically enhance the effectiveness of terrorist tactics. The media, particularly the electronic ones, provide terrorist groups with the large, captive audiences without which their tactics are rendered ineffective. In addition, the salient and dramatic portrayal of terrorist incidents by the media may elicit a process of modeling and imitation. It may be suggested, therefore, that the recent proliferation of terrorist activity is not entirely due to the existence of more or more compelling root causes. Groups' evident preference for the terrorist response is at least partly attributable to the ease with which terrorism can nowadays be exercised, or, as George Will (1979) argued, to the fact that terrorism has become highly "cost-effective."

Summary

In this chapter, the applicability of social psychological theory to the explanation of terrorism has been examined. Assuming that terrorism is a strategy employed by groups to bring about social and political change, its explanation requires answers to two questions. First, what are the conditions that drive groups to seek social and political change? Second, what is the process whereby groups aspiring for such change turn to terrorist violence?

Theories of intergroup conflict, particularly those addressed to the behavior of minority groups, provide a framework within which the first question can be answered. The usefulness of these theories is qualified, however, by examples of terrorist groups that emerged out of privileged majority groups rather than out of disadvantaged minorities. The conditions that lead to the rise of such groups, motivated by ideology rather than by deprivation, have yet to be specified by social psychological theory.

The frustration-aggression and relative deprivation hypotheses comprise the core of answers to the second question. However, in applying these hypotheses to the explanation of terrorism it is essential to consider variations in the nature and intensity of frustrations and deprivations experienced by different groups. The frustrations of West European or North American young radicals are hardly comparable to the plight of national groups that have lost a homeland or been denied sovereignty, or to that of groups suffering religious or ethnic discrimination. In the former case, frustration appears to be insufficiently potent to motivate a mass terrorist movement. Thus, to account for the behavior of the few that do turn to terrorism, it is necessary to take into account personal attributes and dispositions.

The key role that individual factors may play in the dynamics of terrorism sets a limit on the generality of theories that seek to explain it in terms of intergroup processes and conflict. No analysis of minority groups or of intergroup strife in the United States can fully explain the doings of the twelve persons who formed the Symbionese Liberation Army. This is by no means to suggest that social psychological explanations are invalid. Yet it is necessary to recognize the possibility that such explanations might be more valid with respect to some instances of terrorism than to others.

References

Alexander, Y., & Gleason, J. M. (Eds.). (1981). *Behavioral and quantitative perspectives on terrorism*. New York: Pergamon.

Arendt, H. (1973). *Crisis of the republic*. Harmondsworth: Penguin.

Berkowitz, L. (1972). Frustrations, comparisons and other sources of emotional arousal as contributors to social unrest. *Journal of Social Issues, 28,* 77–91.

Billig, M. (1976). *Social psychology and intergroup relations*. London: Academic.

Bonanate, L. (1979). Some unanticipated consequences of terrorism. *Journal of Peace Research, 16,* 195–203.

Bowyer Bell, J. (1978). *A time of terror: How democratic societies respond to revolutionary violence*. New York: Basic Books.

Brown, R. J., & Ross, G. F. (1982). The battle for acceptance: An investigation into the dynamics of intergroup behavior. In H. Tajfel (Ed.), *Social identity and intergroup relations*. Cambridge: Cambridge University Press.

Crenshaw, M. (1981). The causes of terrorism. *Comparative Politics, 14,* 385–397.

Crozier, B. (1960). *The rebels: A study of post-war insurrections*. London: Chatto & Windus.

Davies, J. C. (1962). Toward a theory of revolution. *American Sociological Review, 27,* 5–19.

DeSwaan, A. (1977). Terror as a government service. In M. Hoefnagels (Ed.), *Repression and repressive violence*. Amsterdam: Swets & Zeitlinger.

Devine, P. E., & Rafalko, R. J. (1982). On terror. *The Annals of the American Academy of Political and Social Science, 463,* 39–53.

Dollard, J., Doob, L. W., Miller, N. E., Mowrer, O. H., & Sears, R. R. (1939). *Frustration and aggression*. New Haven: Yale University Press.

Feierabend, I. K., & Feierabend, R. L. (1966). Aggressive behavior within politics, 1948–1962: A cross-national survey. *Journal of Conflict Resolution, 10,* 247–271.

Feierabend, I. K., Feierabend, R. L., & Nesvold, B. A. (1973). The comparative study of revolution and violence. *Comparative Politics, 5,* 393–424.

Ferracuti, F. (1982). A sociopsychiatric interpretation of terrorism. *The Annals of the American Academy of Political and Social Science, 463,* 129–149.

Freedman, L. Z. (1983). Terrorism: Problems of the Polistraxic. In L. Z. Freedman & Y. Alexander (Eds.), *Perspectives on terrorism*. Wilmington: Scholarly Resources.

Fromkin, D. (1975). The strategy of terrorism. *Foreign Affairs, 53,* 683–698.

Gurr, T. R. (1970). *Why men rebel*. Princeton: Princeton University Press.

Hess, H. (1981). Terrorismus and Terrorismus-Diskurs. *Tijdschrift voor Criminologie, 4,* 175–190.

Jenkins, B. M. (1975). International terrorism: A new mode of conflict. In D. Carlton & C. Shaerf (Eds.), *International terrorism and world security*. London: Croom Helm.

Jenkins, B. M. (1983). *Some reflections on recent trends in terrorism* (RAND Paper Series P-6897). Santa Monica: The RAND Corporation.

Kaplan, A. (1981). The psychodynamics of terrorism. In Y. Alexander & J. M. Gleason (Eds.), *Behavioral and quantitative perspectives on terrorism*. New York: Pergamon.

Kielmansegg, P. G. (1978). Politikwissenschaft und Gewaltproblematik. In H. Geissler (Ed.), *Der Weg in die Gewalt*. Munich: Olzog.

Laqueur, W. (1976, March). Terrorism – a balance sheet. *Harper's Magazine,* p. 26.

Lupsha, P. A. (1971). Explanation of political violence: Some psychological theories versus indignation. *Politics and Society, 2,* 89–104.

Marighela, C. (1971). *For the liberation of Brazil*. Harmondsworth: Penguin.

Mickolus, E. F. (1980). *The literature of terrorism*. Westport: Greenwood.

Morf, G. (1970). *Le terrorisme québecois*. Montreal: Editions de l'Homme.

Nagel, W. H. (1980). A socio-legal view on the suppression of terrorism. *International Journal of Sociology of Law, 8,* 218–229.

Paine, L. (1975). *The terrorists*. London: Robert Hale.

Rosenbaum, H. J., & Sederberg, P. C. (1974). Vigilantism: An analysis of establishment violence. *Comparative Politics, 6,* 541–570.

Russell, C. A., Bowman, H., & Miller, H. (1977). Profile of a terrorist. *Military Review, 58,* 24–39.

Schmid, A. P. (1983). *Political terrorism*. Amsterdam: North Holland.

Stohl, M. (1983). *The politics of terrorism*. New York: Dekker.

Tajfel, H. (1981). *Human groups and social categories: Studies in social psychology*. Cambridge: Cambridge University Press.

Thibaut, J., Friedland, N., & Walker, L. (1974) Compliance with rules: Some social determinants. *Journal of Personality and Social Psychology, 30,* 792–801.

Turner, J. C., & Brown, R. J. (1978). Social status, cognitive alternatives, and intergroup relations. In H. Tajfel (Ed.), *Differentiation between social groups: Studies in the social psychology of intergroup relations*. London: Academic.

US Department of State (1983). *Patterns of international terrorism: 1982*. Washington, DC: US Government Printing Office.

Van der Dennen, J. M. G. (1980). *Problems in the concept and definition of aggression, violence, and some related terms*. Groningen: Polemological Institute.

Will, G. (1979). The journalist's role. In B. Netanyahu (Ed.), *Terrorism and the media*. Jerusalem: Jonathan Institute.

Part IV

The Resolution of Conflict

Chapter 7

Bargaining and Arbitration in the Resolution of Conflict

Ian E. Morley, Janette Webb, and Geoffrey M. Stephenson

Introduction

The social psychological literatures concerned with bargaining and with inter-group relations have developed more or less independently. Effectively, there are two bodies of research and theory, with little expression of mutual interest. Consider, for example, Austin and Worchel's (1979) *The Social Psychology of Intergroup Relations*. Neither "negotiation," nor "bargaining," nor "arbitration" appears in the subject index. When negotiation is treated explicitly, little is said about processes of bargaining or arbitration. What is regarded as important is simply the fact that negotiators act as representatives of groups. Thus, they provide paradigm cases of people who perform "boundary roles" (Holmes & Lamm, 1979).

Equally, the literature on negotiation has treated that process more or less independently of the larger structural contexts in which it occurs (Strauss, 1978). A paradigm case is Pruitt's (1981) text, *Negotiation Behavior.* In it Pruitt has attempted to set out a general theory of negotiation, applicable in any context. Effectively, he begins with a statement of *the "bargaining problem"* taken from traditional economic theory. He then presents an abstract analysis of the processes of competition and cooperation by which bargains are made. The result is an individualistic theory in which the process of negotiation is quite literally abstracted from *the intergroup context which gives negotiation its content and point.*

Broadly, what is wrong with the literature on intergroup relations is that it has focused on change, but not considered negotiation as a *mechanism for managing change.* Equally broadly, what is wrong with the literature on negotiation is that it has lost sight of negotiation as a *form of social action,* given meaning by certain structural and social contexts.

This chapter is divided into three related parts. In the first we consider negotiation as a mechanism for managing relations between groups. It is concerned with change, whether actual or potential. We reach three main conclusions. The first is that to understand the process of negotiation we need to ground its study in the context of relations between groups. This means that we must shift the emphasis from models which are individualistic and economic to models which are social and contextual. Second, we conclude that negotiation is to be analyzed as a form of intelligent social action in which participants, individually and collectively, make sense of change, and decide how to manage it. From this point of view, it is important to see the outcomes of negotiation as rules, justified by agreed stories about what has happened and why. Finally, we argue that change is assessed in terms of ideologies derived from interactions within and between groups.

In the second part of the chapter we consider negotiation and arbitration as forms of social conflict. We take the view that arbitration is not so much a judicial procedure as a form of negotiation. Consequently, studies of arbitration may be used to help identify features important to the class of negotiations, considered as a whole. Case material provided by Stephenson and Webb is used to supplement earlier arguments, showing some of the ways in which economic models of bargaining and procedural justice seriously misrepresent the nature of negotiating skill. It is also used to show some of the ways in which bargaining is regulated by administrative norms which artificially narrow its scope.

In the final part of the chapter we conclude that negotiation is one way of writing organizational history. The limits of the process, however, remain to be explored.

The Negotiation of Relations Between Groups

Tajfel (1981) has argued that "the social setting of intergroup relations contributes to making ... individuals what they are and they in turn produce this social setting; they and it develop and change symbiotically." (p. 31). The primary task of a theory of intergroup relations is to explain the nature of the symbiosis.

Tajfel's major contribution to the theory of intergroup relations has been to show that certain kinds of theories – those which are *individualistic* – cannot do this job. In his view they provide inadequate models of people, processes, and contexts: they distort the psychology of the individual because they fail to give him or her "the respect due to a member of a species that created its own environment and its own complexities" (Tajfel, 1981, p. 37); they distort the nature of social processes because they fail to understand how collective cognitive images are created and changed; they distort the nature of social contexts because they fail to say which aspects are important, and why. By default, the social context is assumed to be an "homogeneous medium of freely floating individual particles" (p. 50). It is therefore possible to treat relations between groups as if they involved only relations between individuals.

It is probably fair to say that the work of Tajfel and his associates has provided the major input to European work on intergroup relations. Put simply, they argue that individuals learn what it is to be a member of a group by comparing themselves socially with members of other groups. The major claim made is that relations beween groups are determined by processes of social competition in which each group seeks an identity (as a group) which is positive, distinctive, and secure. The fundamental problems of intergroup relations are thus seen as problems of differentiation between groups (Tajfel, 1978, 1981, 1982; Turner & Giles, 1981). This has been explored in two different contexts. First, there are cases in which groups make claims "based on their right to decide to be different (preserve their separateness) as defined *in their own terms*" (Tajfel, 1981, p.317; italics added). Here the primary focus has been upon low-status groups who are unwilling to work within institutional frameworks controlled by members of a dominant elite. It has involved the analysis of intergroup relations considered as social movements (Morley 1982a; Tajfel, 1981). In such cases it is assumed that certain issues are, and must remain, non-negotiable. For example, Chalmers and Cormick (1971) take the view that negotiation is a power struggle which functions to redistribute services, resources, and opportunities: it does not function to *redistribute power*. If they are correct, basic shifts in power will only occur when minority groups implement change, with or without majority support. Thus, to bring about radical change dissident communities have to act (implement non-negotiable demands) rather than talk about acting (negotiate within the framework of the status quo).

Second, there are cases in which groups are willing to make claims within existing arrangements (Brown, 1978; Louche, 1982). Typically, it is agreed that certain issues are legitimate matters for joint regulation. It is assumed that the method of joint regulation is a process of collective bargaining, and that the parties are negotiating to reach agreements (Morley, 1981a).

Writers on intergroup relations have paid much more attention to the first kind of case than to the second. Tajfel, for example, has more or less ignored the behavior of leaders, or others, meeting face to face to negotiate as representatives of groups (Tajfel, 1981, p.293). Reasons for such neglect are not hard to find. Some writers have stated explicitly that a focus on negotiation is too narrow, given a perspective on social movements (Apfelbaum, 1979; Brown & Ross, 1982; Tajfel, 1981). They mean that the process is conservative in the sense that what goes on the agenda is controlled by members of the dominant group. Others have argued that existing theories of negotiation are individualistic in the sense outlined above (Billig, 1976; Louche, 1982); that is, they treat negotiation as "an isolated and self-sufficient phenomenon" (Louche, 1982, p.480).

Negotiation as a Solution to the Bargaining Problem

Louche has two major criticisms of current social psychological approches to negotiation. Both relate to the origins of such work in economic statements of the "bargaining problem" (Bacharach & Lawler, 1981; Pruitt, 1981; Walton & McKersie, 1965). Such models more or less ignore the effects of social contexts. That is, they attempt abstract analyses which begin from the premise that issues have already been defined. Further, the dynamics of negotiation are reduced to the individual choice of competitive or cooperative tactics. Choices of this kind determine a sequence of bid and counterbid, halting at the point where concessions converge. This is the "solution" to the bargaining problem.

It is fair to say that theories of this kind are individualistic, in Tajfel's (1981) sense. First, they distort the psychology of the individual because they take the character of conflict for granted. It is assumed that issues have already been defined. However, if we are to treat negotiation as a species of intelligent social activity we need to explore the ways in which negotiators work out what is going on, and why (Morley, 1986). Second, such theories distort the process of negotiation. It is much more than a sequence of bid and counterbid. It is a social process in which collective cognitive images are created and changed, as Tajfel's analysis would imply. Specifically, negotiation is part of an historical process in which there is something to argue about. In addition, negotiators are subject to constraints produced by previous commitments (Morley, 1982b; Strauss, 1978). Accordingly, their major task is to find a *formula* linking what is happening now to what has happened in the past, and to what will happen in the future (Kanter, 1984; Zartman, 1977). Once a formula has been found the participants know the general form an agreement will take, and why: the rest is detail. Finally, the theories distort the nature of the social context. They treat it as given, rather than constructed; they fail to show what has historical significance and what has not; and they ignore peoples' theories of social order and social change (Morley, 1986; Strauss, 1978). Instead, it is assumed to be sufficient to say whether contextual factors are likely to increase cooperation or competition between the sides (for whatever reasons).

It is clear that "the process of negotiation needs to be redefined," as Louche (1982) says. One possibility is to consider negotiation as the process by which social order is constructed.

The Construction of Social Order

Economic models regard negotiation as a mechanism for resolving conflicts. This is probably a mistake. It is better to say that negotiation is a mechanism for *managing change*. We assume that the negotiators view change in ways which reflect the values and interests of those they represent. We assume, also, that they manage the change by working out *rules,* regulating the nature of relations between groups (setting out the terms on which the groups will do business). There is thus a clear sense in which negotiators are agents of change, engaged in *writing organizational history* (Morley, 1986; Kanter 1984). We shall consider each of these points in turn.

Negotiation and Problem Solving

Negotiation begins when people recognize and respond to *issues* about relations within and between groups. These concern change, or the possibility of change, in an existing social order. Changes of this kind pose problems because they are inherently ambiguous (Morley, 1986) and because they cannot be completely described (Bennett & Feldman, 1981).

The problem of ambiguity arises because "almost any act can be associated with diverse causes, effects, and meanings" (Bennett & Feldman, 1981). The obvious answer is to say that people are able to work out what is going on, and why, because they have organized systems of values, attitudes, and beliefs (that is, ideologies). It has long been recognized that a central task of a theory of group relations is to show how such perceptions derive from social interactions within and between groups (Sherif & Sherif, 1969; Tajfel, 1981; Turner & Giles, 1981).

Problems of the complexity of social action have received much less consideration in the literature. To quote Bennett and Feldman (1981), what matters is that

social actions are so complex that exhaustive descriptions are impossible ... Most important, the meaning of an action has little or no connection to the sheer quantity of detail in accounts about it. Constructing an interpretation for problematic social action ... requires the use of some communications device that simplifies the natural event, selects out a set of information about it, symbolises the information in some way, and organizes it so that the adjudicators can make an unambiguous interpretation and judge its validity. (pp. 66–67)

Bennett and Feldman argue that *stories* are "the most elegant and widely used communication devices for these purposes" (p. 67). Other writers have utilized the notion of a script (Gioia & Poole, 1984). The differences between these accounts are not important for our purposes. What is important is that change, actual or potential, is linked to *paradigm cases which illustrate threats and opportunities, and how they might be handled.* The threats are threats to the values of groups. The opportunities are opportunities to pursue the values of groups. The paradigm cases bring into focus beliefs about ends and means which help to define negotiators' identities as representatives of groups (Morley, 1982a, 1986). This shows one of the ways in which the literature on negotiation can supplement the literature on intergroup relations.

It is worth noting also that scripts are not imposed, nor are they permanent (Hosking & Morley, 1985). Endorsement of a script and action based upon it are the results of a process of intragroup bargaining in which different people try out different arguments, and sponsor different scripts. There are, therefore, two further reasons why research on bargaining is important to research on intergroup relations. The literature suggests that the decision to proceed with negotiations between groups is itself the result of negotiations within groups (Lockhart, 1979; Mitchell, 1981; Morley, 1981b, 1982b; Walton & McKersie, 1965; Warr, 1973), and that differentiation within groups may be much more important than writers such as Tajfel have supposed (Morley, 1982a; Stephenson, 1981, 1984).

Warr's (1973) study of collective bargaining suggests that a period of intra-group conflict (which he calls breaking up) is an almost inevitable feature of negotiation between groups. In some cases the conflict is so severe that important decisions cannot be made: negotiation between the groups loses momentum, or breaks down altogether. One effect may be the modification of party positions, as new scripts (or themes) come to the fore. This has led to the suggestion that there are no fixed positions in negotiation. The suggestion is important, but it is not entirely true, as Mitchell (1981) has pointed out. Party positions are sometimes the result of intraorganizational bargaining which has been protracted and complex. In such cases the balance of forces within the group will be extremely difficult to change. The group will be frozen, in Lewin's terms (Lewin, 1948). Changes in position which imply a renewal of competition within the group may be avoided "at almost any cost" (Mitchell, 1981, p. 328).

Negotiation as social history

When we say that negotiators are writing organizational history we are treating negotiation as a form of conflict in which parties jointly decide how to handle issues as they arise in particular social contexts. What is crucial is not that the negotiators reach agreements (resolving the conflict) but that the agreements can be *justified as rules,* defining the terms on which the parties will do business. This is a further reason why the story metaphor is important. One outcome of negotiation is frequently an agreed story about what has happened, and why. That is to say, outcomes of negotiation may be described as reports about the past designed to elicit the present actions required for the future (Kanter, 1984; Morley, 1986). There is therefore one fundamental reason why the study of negotiation should not be abstracted from the historical contexts in which it occurs: *it is a process by which that context is constructed* (Hosking & Morley, 1985).

In general, intergroup relations occur because people have *projects,* based in their membership of different groups. Social action is an attempt to identify possible projects; to choose between them; and to get others to "fit in" with projects of one's own (Athay & Darley, 1981). There are two sides to this activity. One is *cognitive:* negotiators are trying to work out *intellectually* what is happening, and why. (It is also social, because it may itself be the result of negotiation within a group [Morley, 1986; Steinbruner, 1977; Weick, 1979]). The other is *political:* people with different levels of motivation, commitment, power potential, and skill are trying to establish what is acceptable or viable in a given context. Thus, to understand intergroup relations is to understand those individual and collective processes by which group members *make sense* of what is going on, and why, and what should be done. It is to understand those processes which give intergroup relations their meaning and point.

Taken together, the above two sections suggest that, if we are to give negotiators the respect they are due, we need to treat negotiation as an example of *intelligent social action.*

Negotiation and Arbitration as Forms of Social Conflict

We are concerned with those kinds of negotiation, or collective bargaining, in which negotiators represent organizational or institutional groups. Specifically, we shall examine cases arbitrated by third parties.

It is usual to draw distinctions between different kinds of third party intervention. Conciliation and mediation are processes in which the third party takes an advisory role. Arbitration is closer to a formal judicial review in which decision making is handed to the third party, sometimes freely (voluntary arbitration), sometimes not (compulsory arbitration).

We believe that the study of third-party intervention is important for three reasons. First, it brings certain aspects of direct negotiation into sharper focus. Second, it helps to ground the study of direct negotiations in the wider context of relations between groups. Third, it suggests that the psychological similarities between direct negotiation, conciliation, mediation, and arbitration may be much more important than the differences.

Douglas' classic studies of mediation have suggested some of the ways in which this kind of analysis may proceed (Douglas, 1957, 1962; Morley & Stephenson, 1977; Webb, 1985a). Here, we hope to extend the analysis using the case studies of arbitration set out by Stephenson and Webb (1984) and Webb (1982; 1985a, b).

Stephenson and Webb's Case Studies of Arbitration

The cases described by Stephenson and Webb (1984) all concern the presentation of arguments to third parties who are asked to resolve the dispute. All deal with aspects of British industrial relations. Some describe disputes between an individual and an employer; others describe collective disputes between managements and trades unions. The individual disputes are claims of unfair dismissal submitted to industrial tribunals (ITs; records are available at the Central Office of Industrial Tribunals, London). The collective disputes are arbitrations conducted by the Advisory Conciliation and Arbitration Service (ACAS) or by the Central Arbitration Committee (CAC). A description of these institutions and their place in British industrial relations is given in Dickens (1969).

In the individual cases the IT has to decide whether the individual was treated fairly or not. In the collective cases arbitrators have to deal with a very wide range of terms and conditions of employment. However, where the cases submitted to ACAS may be described as *ad hoc,* the cases submitted to the CAC are framed in terms of employment legislation (typically concerned with fair wages or the disclosure of information to trade unions for collective bargaining).

The cases described by Webb (1982) represent the final stage of the disputes procedure in public sector negotiations between management and unions.

We wish to discuss four main themes which emerge from these kinds of cases: negotiation as story telling, arbitration considered as procedural justice, bargaining style, and the role of the arbitrator.

Negotiation as Story Telling

Arbitrators have to work out what has happened in a particular case, and why. They have also to decide what should be done. Some accounts make the activity of the arbitrator look rather like a process of deductive reasoning from straightforward premises (Thibaut & Walker, 1975). The cases reported in Stephenson and Webb (1984) suggest, however, that the arbitrator must construct a story with a clear structure on the basis of reasoning which is partisan and highly stylized; dramatizing what has happened in the past and what will happen in the future. Thus, he or she must recognize that the evidence provided is more or less arbitrary (see Cicourel, 1976). The reasoning is only partly deductive, and the cases are not at all straightforward.

Apparently, the adversarial nature of the proceedings produces effects similar to those observed in other judicial or quasi-judicial contexts. Bennett and Feldman describe the process of a trial in the following terms.

Each side misses, or chooses to ignore, some potentially important aspect of the incident in question ... Both sides struggle to redefine facts consistently in the direction that best establishes their competing claims about the incident. These struggles over facts, definitions, and interpretations become the hard substance for judgment. In almost any trial there is the uneasy possibility that neither case captures the subtle reality of the incident. (1981, p.93)

This is one reason it is important to have arbitrators who have detailed knowledge of an institution or an industry, who know how such accounts might be assembled.

Two further points are of general significance. The first concerns the analysis of adversarial procedures in legal or quasi-legal contests: namely, that judicial or quasi-judicial procedures involve much more than the straightforward presentation and examination of facts. This is why we have followed Cicourel (1976) and called certain features of the process arbitrary. We believe that current social psychological models of procedural justice (Thibaut & Walker, 1975; Walker & Lind, 1984) have failed sufficiently to appreciate the partisan, stylized, dramatic reasoning which constitutes the *struggle* over facts, definitions, and interpretations. Consequently, the study of procedural justice has proceeded independently of the study of relations between groups. As we shall see, what is lacking is an appreciation of the social significance of social institutions.

The second point concerns the nature of the process of negotiation. The study of arbitration hightlights the fact that, typically, negotiation is an adversary procedure in which participants face problems of ambiguity and complexity (Morley, 1982, 1986; Winham, 1977). Negotiators, like arbitrators, create order by reconstructing a story from reports which are partisan and incomplete. They use this story as a basis for making a judgment.

If Bennett and Feldman (1981) are correct, the story provides the basis for action because it connects actors and actions "through a consistent set of purposes, agencies, and scenes" (p. 95). This may be the basis of a formula which will be an effective guide to action. The formula will be implemented to the extent that it is understood, and seen as viable, given the power of the parties to control the issues concerned.

Arbitration Considered as Procedural Justice

The theory of procedural justice set out by Thibaut, Walker, and Lind (Thibaut & Walker, 1975; Walker & Lind, 1984) asserts that, given conflicts of interest, the "goal of the dispute resolution process must be the allocation of outcomes in line with disputant standards for fairness" (Walker & Lind, 1984, p. 307). According to the theory, the predominant standards are those described in equity theory. In other words, third parties will attempt to establish an equitable outcome, defined in terms of the profits, investments, and expected outcomes of the individuals or groups. Analysis of the cases set out by Stephenson and Webb (1984) shows that, at best, this is only part of the story. It fails to show how different institutions have different views about what makes a dispute amenable to arbitration. It also ignores the fact that different administrative arrangements lead to different rules of evidence, so to speak.

Arbitration requires issues to be defined in ways which allow the arbitrator to decide. This happens in different ways in different institutions. That is to say, different institutions use different *conventions* to determine the facts of a case. Those used by the ITs meant that, typically, the employer had to show, first, that there was "good reason" for the dismissal; second, that there was reasonable evidence on which to base the dismissal; and third, that he (or she) had followed some consistent procedure. The cases submitted to ACAS contained a wide range of issues. However, the conventions used meant that issues became narrowly defined, so that a third party could make a "factual" decision, almost in yes/no terms. In the CAC cases the disputes were defined in terms of employment legislation. Claims about fair pay required the arbitrator to assess the relative position of one group compared with others. In the majority of cases, establishing a claim meant a series of clear-cut steps which allowed a more or less precisely calculated solution to the inherently vague concept of fair wages. Explicit appeals to fairness, or equity, were rare. Claims about disclosure of information were most often attempts to establish the right to bargain. In the short term they were about the relative status of the parties. A few claims were presented as collaborative. The employer agreed that a group of employees was in an unfavorable position. The object of the exercise was to find a way round restrictions in funding imposed by central government. This was, perhaps, a way of protecting the bargaining relationship between union and management: uniting against a "common enemy," namely, the government.

Arbitration works to narrow the focus of the participants. It is organized around surface issues. Whether these have wider significance may never be discussed. In the case of the tribunals this seems to have occurred because the tribunals adopted an "efficiency" rather than a "welfare" orientation. They created an administrative concept of fairness which allowed them efficiently to dispose of cases. Once the employer succeeded in telling the right kind of story, he or she was defined as acting reasonably. Accordingly, the case could be settled. The tribunal could move on to the next. The result was a set of procedures in which the perspective of the individual applicant became secondary to that of the employer. In particular, little or no attempt was made to explore the sense of grievance or victimization evident in applicants' written statements. Once a practice was accepted as standard, there was little opportunity to explore its value as a practice. (Consider, for example, the case of a black temporary employee who was attempting to move to a permanent post. The move was contingent upon the result of a medical examination. The applicant was asked to produce a passport and birth certificate before the examination. He felt that this represented a special condition, to which he objected. The tribunal, however, accepted this as standard treatment, and therefore "fair." They dismissed the claim. There was no attempt to question the need for such a procedure only in the case of black applicants.) There was a narrowing of focus in the collective contexts, also. The need to establish a case worked closely to delineate the areas of dispute. Parties, particularly the trades unions, set limited goals, precisely stated. This is by no means the norm in direct bargaining between the parties (Morley, 1981a, b; Snyder & Diesing, 1977).

Walton and McKersie (1965) make a distinction between distributive and integrative bargaining. The former deals with *issues* about the distribution of gains and losses in a fixed sum game. The latter deals with *problems,* defined as areas of joint concern, located within a variable sum game. In distributive bargaining the parties know what they want, place those items on the agenda, and use struggle tactics (pressure bargaining) to achieve their goals (McKersie & Hunter, 1973; Pruitt, 1971). Issues are identified explicitly and dealt with "surgically" one by one (McKersie & Hunter, 1973, p. 161). Integrative bargaining is quite different. McKersie and Hunter (1973) say it involves an indirect approach. The agenda is not determined unilaterally, but arises from an exercise in problem definition and problem solving, jointly undertaken. Consequently, related problems can be considered as a whole, with the parties cooperating in their solution. In this sense the bargaining process integrates the parties, however temporary the accommodation. The distinction between the two kinds of bargaining is complex and needs to be used with caution. It may be useful, however, in the present context. What we have seen, in Walton and McKersie's terms, is a tendency for arbitration to convert problems into issues. That is to say, arbitration is structured in ways which inhibit the development of integrative bargaining processes. In this respect the cases we have described are very like the cases which go through other kinds of formal procedure (Clegg, 1979; Hyman, 1972).

Bargaining Style

It is commonplace to classify bargaining styles as essentially cooperative or essentially competitive. It is assumed that people are fundamentally cooperatively or competitively disposed, although their behavior may be modified by the behavior of the other, and by changes in negotiating arrangements (Druckman, 1977; Raven & Rubin, 1983; Rubin & Brown, 1975). What emerges from the cases, rather, is that bargaining style is a matter of strategy, to be construed as a method of structuring interaction in ways that enhance a group's strengths and minimize its weaknesses. It is thus to be analyzed in the kind of way that Biggart (1981) has analyzed President Reagan's leadership style: in terms of the nature of relationships rather than in terms of the dispositions of an individual.

Given the constraints imposed by the framework of procedure, or arbitration, the primary job of the negotiator is to win the case. Bound by conventions which confine conflict to a small number of issues, narrowly defined, his or her first job is to recognize these constraints and work within them.

This means working with the arguments made available by the context. It may be said that the participants in the CAC forum studied by Stephenson and Webb (1984) were dealing with the distribution of resources, narrowly defined. However, what counted as a resource was dependent upon what the legislation allowed as legitimate matters for bargaining. In public sector bodies, for example, the union could argue that a noncontributory pension fund was necessary as part of the fair wage, given that comparable civil service employees had such a scheme.

Even if issues are narrowly defined, however, they may be brought to the fore in more than one way. One of the skills of negotiation is to raise issues in ways which recognize they are part of an historical process of change. In this respect it is important that arbitration is seen not only as the last stage in a disputes procedure, but also as the starting point for future negotiation. The subtlety of strategy can be quite surprising, even in simple cases. In one case, for example, drivers of car transporters discovered that their company had been paying more favorable bonuses to drivers from another depot. This had been going on for 7 years. The company had privately conceded that the situation would not be allowed to continue. The union wished to claim what the drivers saw as 7 years' back payment of lost bonuses. Accordingly, the dispute went to arbitration as an argument about the normal capacity of the lorries. The argument was not based on appeals to fairness and social justice. It was rather a technical case, based on statistics, figures, talk about technological limits, and so on. Its function was not to resolve one conflict but to begin another.

Aspects such as these are difficult to capture in individualistic accounts such as those of Raven and Rubin (1983). Indeed, it is almost a defining feature of such analyses that they concentrate upon the form of negotiation rather than its content. They are not interested in what the arguments mean.

The Role of the Arbitrator

In the cases considered by Stephenson and Webb, the third party may be considered as representing a standard of good practice in industrial relations. The third parties themselves are also committed to an authority: to the body they represent, and indirectly to the government. Consequently, they find collaborative claims particularly diffcult (they may, after all, result in legitimation of a claim in opposition to a stance taken by government).

Pressures of this kind have been identified by writers such as McGrath (1966). Nevertheless, few treatments give due recognition to the fact that the arbitrator *is a strategic actor in his (or her) own right, representing different interests and concerns according to the wider political context.* Instead, much of the literature assumes a concession-convergence model of negotiation. This implies that third parties accept the dispute at face value and leads to a view of arbitration as a face-saving device, or as a threat to be used in inducing faster concessions from the parties: the arbitrator is not there to change the nature of the bargaining process, but to manage the process of convergence upon a settlement point which the parties would like, but would be hesitant to propose (Pruitt, 1971; Webb, 1982). Webb (1982) has argued that such a view is more appropriate to cases which are simple rather than complex.

One arbitration board has described the problems of complexity in the following terms:

We have been presented with two claims which have not been advanced on the same basis. They have also produced different responses from the other parties concerned with the outcome of our decision. As a result we have been faced with four divergent views of the problems and events ... together with incompatible suggestions for dealing with them. (Webb, 1985, p.6)

Complexity of case has three main implications for the role of the arbitrator. First, arbitrators have sometimes felt it wise only to indicate the general direction in which they felt the parties should travel (Webb, 1982, p.196). They are thus providing a framework, rather than a definitive answer to the dispute. The details of the implementation are to be the subject of future negotiations between the sides.

Second, it is clear from Webb's (1982) data that as cases become more complex arbitrators become more involved as third *parties,* with specific interests and distinctive points of view. They develop their own theories about the root causes of disputes which appear in a series of references (e. g., that they are due to an industry's lack of a systematic job evaluation and grading scheme). This means that they are sometimes willing to make quite extensive recommendations on the regulation of industrial relations within an industry. There is thus a clear sense in which Webb's (1982) data support Downs' (1957) view that complexity promotes ideology in decision making.

Third, as cases become more complex it is especially important that the arbitrator makes a clear distinction between interpersonal and interparty climates, or stages, in negotiation (Stephenson, 1984; Webb, 1982). Field studies of research on stages in negotiation have derived from a theoretical perspective in which interpersonal and interparty concerns have been seen as orthogonal dimensions, running from high to low, in each case (Morley, 1982a; Stephenson, 1981, 1984). This contrasts with the position of Tajfel and his associates in which they form opposite ends of a continuum. It is argued that the interpersonal stage allows the parties unofficially to reconnoiter the bargaining range (Douglas, 1957, 1962). In this context it allows the arbitrator to initiate the creative work necessary to find a solution and sell it to the parties concerned.

The idea that creativity shows phase changes in conflict episodes deserves further study. One interesting line of development has been initiated by Hare (1985), who has adapted Bales & Cohen's (1979) SYMLOG methodology to study protest demonstrations, a resettlement project, conflicts between ethnic groups, and the Camp David summit. In some cases what is immediately apparent is the search for "images, themes, plots, or scripts on which all parties can agree" (Hare, 1985, p.83). Presumably, these help polarized individuals to unify their perceptual fields, finding social identities which have significant elements in common. In other cases it is evident that conflict has been managed by manipulating the composition of the negotiation team, effectively forming subcommittees or drafting groups and excluding the members who were most dominant (although not necessarily the most hardline, Hare, 1985, pp.138–139).

Arbitration may be seen as an institution for limiting the scale of conflict by confining it to narrow issues, avoiding open-ended commitments to the solution of broad problems. This sort of analysis is important, as we have shown. However, it is also important not to forget that arbitration is also a social process which derives its significance from a wider context – in this case, that of industrial relations. Thus, the choice of arbitrator and the principles applied in reaching a decision are an important basis for dispute in their own right (Hyman, 1972; Webb, 1982).

In some cases arbitration boards begin to assume an influential role in deciding industrial relations policies. To the extent that their recommendations are far-reaching, they will find that related issues will be referred to them for further consideration. Let us repeat that arbitration thus ceases to be the end point of a dispute. Rather it becomes one part of a much longer *cycle* of negotiation which results in a series of changes in the industry. Consequently, the decisions of the board become contentious issues in themselves (Webb, 1982): the parties may disagree about the wider implications of such decisions, or negotiate how they are to be implemented in practice, or they may refer issues back to arbitration in a slightly altered form.

Discussion and Conclusions

Arbitration, and disputes procedures generally, institutionalize conflict. They do not resolve conflict so much as regulate it (Batstone, 1969; Deutsch, 1973). They do this largely by defining the conflict as a finite technical problem. Part of the art (or artifice) of the bargainer is in finding a way of expressing conflict in terms which are concrete and amenable to arbitration. Hence, much of the work of the bargainers takes place before the parties come together. It is vested in the statement of the issues. Hyman (1982) has described the social situation which is created as artificial. Certainly, a set of administrative norms are evolved through legislation and social practice, defining what conflict can be about and what the third party can do. This is, perhaps, most evident in the cases submitted to the CAC. These were explicitly about fairness. But explicit appeals to fairness or equity were rare. Rather, the process was managed by applying a set of technical rules. Those who understood the rules were more likely to be successful negotiators than those who did not.

There are obvious advantages to this form of practice (Batstone, 1969). The disadvantages are related to the difficulty of addressing the underlying issues directly. This occurs rarely, perhaps only in complex cases. It may be important also to distinguish between formal and informal conferences (Clegg, 1979; Hyman, 1982). Hyman (1982) has noted that cases are settled informally, after the parties have registered a failure to agree. As he says, "Procedural discussions may reveal dimensions of a problem which are not encompassed by the terms of reference and cannot appropriately be resolved in the formal setting" (Hyman, 1982, p. 60). Clegg (1979) regards the distinction between formal and informal kinds of bargaining as so important that he treats it as a defining attribute of bargaining styles. Both Clegg (1979) and Hyman (1982) argue that informality favors the development of integrative bargaining. Nevertheless, integrative bargaining is relatively rare: most bargaining is distributive bargaining over issues (Anthony, 1977; McKersie & Hunter, 1973; Morley, 1981b).

Strauss (1978) has treated integrative bargaining under the heading of "building cooperative structures". His account of the negotiations dealing with the economic union of the Benelux countries, Belgium, Luxembourg, and the Netherlands, is of particular interest. He notes that competition between the parties was played down because the benefits of such a union were seen as an "overriding common stake" (p. 160). The negotiations were overt, technical, complex, linked, multiple and sequential. The negotiators gained considerable experience of working together. They were backed up by teams of experts who carried out research and held inquiries. We may suppose that without contextual conditions of this kind integrative bargaining (cooperative negotiation) is likely to be relatively brief and limited in scope.

What is more important, perhaps, is that negotiators develop close, informal bargaining relationships with members of the other side: if they are to solve problems they may have to do so by building special relationships with opponents, possibly collusive in character (Batstone, Boraston, & Frenkel, 1977; Stephenson, 1981, 1984).

Some writers make a clear distinction between arbitration, which they see as a judicial process, and negotiation, which they do not. The distinction seems tenable only in simple cases in which it is relatively easy for the arbitrator to give answers in yes/no terms. Even then it is worth noting that the negotiators have to make the award work by telling appropriate stories about what has happened, and why. The power to make a decision is not the same as the power to make it stick, as Burns (1978) has shown. In more complex cases the hearings are multiparty negotiations in which the arbitration board may take a powerful and creative role as a party in its own right (Webb, 1982).

Arbitration, mediation, conciliation, and negotiation are exercises in writing organizational history. They are themselves forms of relations between groups. The outcomes are rules, justified by reconstructing what has happened in the past, and why (Kanter, 1984). This is why the study of negotiation can contribute to the study of relations within and between groups. It is also why "a social psychology without a full focus on history is a blind social psychology" (Strauss, 1959, p. 173).

If we wish to locate the study of negotiation more precisely within the study of group relations there are (at least) two jobs which need to be done. First, we need to consider the limits of negotiation to see just how much history can be written in this way. If Strauss (1978) is correct, the answer is not obvious. His own review, explicitly designed to cover a wide range of negotiations and contexts, suggests that

what someone takes as limits to negotiation – in any given situation – may not really constitute limits. Given more resources of any kind ... – time, money, skill, information, "awareness," boldness, or perhaps desperation – given that, what were previously taken as non-negotiable [issues] may in fact be negotiable in some sense, some way, some degree. Whether or not that is so has to be discovered, not merely assumed ... I only say that the limits require exploration. (p. 259)

This should be a major task of research on relations between groups. To complete it we shall have to take seriously the idea that the skills of the participants form an important resource. They also form an important part of the social context (Hosking & Morley, 1985).

A second major task is further to examine the compulsions and pressures which operate within and between groups. When we know more about actors' views of the problems and challenges they face (and how these views are learned) we will be able to say much more about the nature of negotiation considered as a species of intelligent social action (Morley, 1986). We will also be in a better position to integrate the literature on negotiation with the literature on leadership (Brown & Hosking, in press; Hosking & Morley, 1985; Morley & Hosking, 1985) and other decisions relating to conflict between groups (Chalmers & Cormick, 1971; Hartley, Kelly, & Nicholson, 1983).

References

Anthony, P. D. (1977). *The conduct of industrial relations*. London: Institute of Personnel Management.

Apfelbaum, E. (1979). Relations of dominantion and movements for liberation: An analysis of power between groups. In W. G. Austin & S. Worchel (Eds.), *The social psychology of intergroup relations*. Monterey, CA: Brooks/Cole.

Athay, M., & Darley, J. M. (1981). Toward an interaction-centered theory of personality. In

N. Cantor & J. W. Kihlstrom (Eds.), *Personality, cognition, and social behavior.* Hillsdale, NJ: Erlbaum.

Austin, W. G., & Worchel, S. (Eds.). (1979). *The social psychology of intergroup relations.* Monterey, CA: Brooks/Cole.

Bacharach, S. P., & Lawler, E. J. (1981). *Bargaining: Power, tactics, and outcomes.* San Francisco: Jossey-Bass.

Bales, R. F., & Cohen, S. P. (with Williamson, S. A.) (1979). *SYMLOG: A system for the multiple level observation of groups.* New York: Free Press.

Batstone, E. (1969). The organization of conflict. In G. M. Stephenson & C. J. Brotherton (Eds.), *Industrial relations: A social psychological approach.* Chichester: Wiley.

Batstone, E., Boraston, I., & Frenkel, S. (1977). *Shop stewards in action.* Oxford: Blackwell.

Bennett, W. L., & Feldman, M. S. (1981). *Reconstructing reality in the courtroom.* London: Tavistock.

Biggart, N. W. (1981). Management style as strategic interaction: the case of President Reagan. *The Journal of Applied Behavioral Science, 17,* 291–308.

Billig, M. (1976). *Social psychology and intergroup relations.* London: Academic.

Brown, H., & Hosking, D. M. (in press). Distributed leadership and skilled performance as successful organization in social movements. *Human Relations.*

Brown, R. J. (1978). Divided we fall: An analysis of relations between sections of a factory workforce. In H. Tajfel (Ed.), *Differentiation between social groups: Studies in the social psychology of intergroup relations.* London: Academic.

Brown, R. J., & Ross, G. F. (1982). The battle for acceptance: An investigation into the dynamics of intergroup behaviour. In H. Tajfel (Ed.), *Social identity and intergroup relations.* Cambridge: Cambridge University Press.

Burns, J. M. (1978). *Leadership.* New York: Harper & Row.

Chalmers, W. E., & Cormick, G. W. (Eds.). (1971). *Racial conflict and negotiations: Perspective and first case studies.* Ann Arbor: Institute of Labor and Industrial Relations: The University of Michigan and the National Center for Dispute Settlement of the American Arbitration Association.

Cicourel, A. (1976). *The social organization of juvenile justice.* London: Heinemann.

Clegg, H. A. (1979). *The changing system of industrial relations in Great Britain.* Oxford: Blackwell.

Deutsch, M. (1973). *The resolution of conflict: Constructive and destructive processes.* New Haven: Yale University Press.

Dickens, L. (1969). Conciliation, mediation, and arbitration in British industrial relations. In G. M. Stephenson, & C. J. Brotherton (Eds.), *Industrial relations: A social psychological approach.* Chichester: Wiley.

Douglas, A. (1957). The peaceful settlement of industrial and intergroup disputes. *Journal of Conflict Resolution, 1,* 69–81.

Douglas, A. (1962). *Industrial peacemaking.* New York: Columbia Univeristy Press.

Downs, A. (1957). *An economic theory of democracy.* New York: Harper & Row.

Druckman, D. (Ed.). (1977). *Negotiations: Social psychological perspectives.* Beverly Hills: Sage.

Gioia, D., & Poole, P. P. (1984). Scripts in organisational behavior. *Academy of Management Review, 2,* 449–459.

Hare, A. P. (1985). *Social interaction as drama: Applications from conflict resolution.* Beverly Hills: Sage.

Hartley, J., Kelly, J., & Nicholson N. (1983). *Steel strike: A case study in industrial relations.* London: Batsford.

Holmes, J. G., & Lamm, H. (1979). Boundary roles and the reduction of conflict. In W. G. Austin, & S. Worchel (Eds.), *The social psychology of intergroup relations.* Monterey, CA: Brooks/Cole.

Hosking, D. M., & Morley, I. E. (1985). The skills of leadership. Paper presented at 8th Biennial Leadership Symposium, Texas Tech University, Lubbock, Texas, USA, 23–27 July.

Hosking, D. M., & Morley, I. E. (1986). Leadership and organization: processes of influence, negotiation, and exchange. Working paper, Department of Psychology, University of Warwick.

Hyman, R. (1972). *Disputes procedure in action.* London: Heinemann.

Kanter, R. (1984). *The change masters: Corporate entrepreneurs at work.* London: Allen & Unwin.

Lewin, K. (1948). *Resolving social conflicts.* New York: Harper.

Lockhart, C. (1979). *Bargaining in international conflicts.* New York: Columbia University Press.

Louche, C. (1982). Open conflict and the dynamics of intergroup negotiations. In H. Tajfel (Ed.), *Social identity and intergroup relations.* Cambridge: Cambridge University Press.

McGrath, J. E. (1966). A social psychological approach to the study of negotiation. In R. Bowers (Ed.), *Studies on behavior in organizations: A research symposium.* Athens, GA: University of Georgia Press.

McKersie, R. B., & Hunter, L. C. (1973). *Pay, productivity and collective bargaining.* London: Macmillan.

Mitchell, C. R. (1981). *The structure of international conflict.* London: Macmillan.

Morley, I. E. (1981a). Negotiation and bargaining. In M. Argyle (Ed.), *Social skills and work.* London: Methuen.

Morley, I. E. (1981b). Bargaining and negotiation. In C. L. Cooper (Ed.), *Psychology and management: A text for managers and trade unionists.* London: Macmillan/The British Psychological Society.

Morley, I. E. (1982a). Henri Tajfel's *Human groups and social categories. British Journal of Social Psychology, 21,* 189-201.

Morley, I. E. (1982b). Preparation for negotiation. In H. Brandstätter, J. H. Davis, G. Stocker-Kreichgauer (Eds.), *Group decision making.* London: Academic.

Morley, I. E. (1986). Negotiating and bargaining. In O. Hargie (Ed.), *A handbook of communication skills.* Beckenham: Croom Helm.

Morley, I. E. & Hosking, D. M. (in press). The skills of leadership. In H.-W. Schroiff, & G. Debus (Eds.), *Proceedings of the West European conference on the psychology of work and organization, Aachen, FRG, 1-3 April 1985.* Amsterdam: North Holland.

Morley, I. E., & Stephenson, G. M. (1977). *The social psychology of bargaining.* London: Allen & Unwin.

Pruitt, D. G. (1971). Indirect communication and the search for agreement in negotiation. *Journal of Applied Social Psychology, 1,* 205-239.

Pruitt, D. G. (1981). *Negotiation behavior.* New York: Academic.

Raven, B. H., & Rubin, J. Z. (1983). *Social psychology.* Chichester: Wiley.

Rubin, J. Z., & Brown, B. R. (1975). *The social psychology of bargaining and negotiation.* New York: Academic.

Sherif, M., & Sherif, C. W. (1969). *Social psychology.* New York: Harper & Row.

Snyder, G. H., & Diesing, P. (1977). *Conflict among nations: Bargaining, decision-making, and system structure in international crises.* Princeton: Princeton University Press.

Steinbruner, J. D. (1977). *The cybernetic theory of decision.* Princeton, NJ: Princeton University Press.

Stephenson, G. M. (1981). Intergroup bargaining and negotiation. In J. C. Turner, & H. Giles (Eds.), *Intergroup behaviour.* Oxford: Blackwell.

Stephenson, G. M. (1984). Intergroup and interpersonal dimensions of bargaining and negotiation. In H. Tajfel (Ed.), *The social dimension,* (Vol. 2). Cambridge: Cambridge University Press.

Stephenson, G. M., & Webb, J. (1984). *Procedures of arbitration.* Report to the Economic and Social Research Council.

Strauss, A. (1959). *Mirrors and masks.* Glencoe: Free Press.

Strauss, A. (1978). *Negotiations: Varieties, contexts, processes and social order.* San Francisco: Jossey-Bass.

Tajfel, H. (Ed.). (1978). *Differentiation between social groups: Studies on the social psychology of intergroup relations.* London: Academic.

Tajfel, H. (1981). *Human groups and social categories.* Cambridge: Cambridge University Press.

Tajfel, H. (Ed.). (1982). *Social identity and intergroup relations.* Cambridge: Cambridge University Press.

Thibaut, J., & Walker, L. (1975). *Procedural justice*. Hillsdale, NJ: Erlbaum.

Turner, J. C., & Giles, H. (Eds.). (1981). *Intergroup behaviour*. Oxford: Blackwell.

Walker, L., & Lind, A. (1984). Psychological studies of procedural models. In G. M. Stephenson, & Davis, J. H. (Eds.), *Progress in applied social psychology,* (Vol. 2). Chichester: Wiley.

Walton, R. E., & McKersie, R. B. (1965). *A behavioral theory of labor negotiations: An analysis of a social interaction system*. New York: McGraw-Hill.

Warr, P. B. (1973). *Psychology and collective bargaining*. London: Hutchinson.

Webb, J. (1982). *Social psychological aspects of third party intervention in industrial disputes*. Doctoral thesis, University of Nottingham.

Webb, J. (1985). The effects of the relative simplicity or complexity of disputes on the process of arbitration in the public sector. Unpublished research paper, Management Centre, University of Aston.

Weick, K. (1979). *The social psychology of organizing*. Reading, MA: Addison-Wesley.

Winham, G. R. (1977). Complexity in international negotiation. In D. Druckman (Ed.), *Negotiations: Social Psychological perspectives*. Beverly Hills: Sage.

Zartman, I. W. (1977). Negotiation as a joint decision-making process. In I. W. Zartman (Ed.), *The negotiation process: Theories and applications*. Beverly Hills: Sage.

Chapter 8

Negotiating with Terrorists

Ariel Merari and Nehemia Friedland

Terrorism has aroused much concern in recent years. Such concern can hardly be attributed to terrorism's physical effects. As a form of warfare, terrorism is probably the least lethal, and as a source of human suffering it undoubtedly trails far behind certain diseases, natural disasters, or man-made problems such as road accidents or common criminal activity. The undeniable impact that terrorism has had on public mood and, in some cases, on government policies has resulted from factors other than its toll in human lives. Most important among these factors is terrorism's ability to undermine government legitimacy as a guardian of public peace and as a trustee of the democratic decision-making process. In this regard, the seizure of hostages and the issuing of demands as a condition for their release is the most effective terrorist tactic.

This chapter examines hostage situations. The first section presents the problem, the dilemmas facing governments, and the major types of hostage incidents. Following the portrayal of the problem, we address in the second section the issue of response. This issue has a strategic and tactical facet. The former refers to the policies that governments may implement in order to prevent politically motivated hostage taking. The tactical facet concerns the management of hostage situations and the conduct of hostage negotiations. Both facets are presented with a view to the identification of issues that lend themselves to psychological and, particularly, social psychological analysis.

The Problem: On the Nature and Types of Hostage Incidents

Although in a sense all terrorism is extortionate, as it attempts to induce political change through intimidation, most terrorist acts do not pose an acute challenge to governments. Terrorist acts such as bombings or assassinations usually do not present a government with an immediate dilemma. In incidents involving hostages, on the other hand, the government faces the choice between its responsibility to safeguard the lives of the hostages and its duty to uphold its policy principles. Any course of action has its own political risks, and the choices, therefore, are always painful and bound to be criticized by some segments of the public. Typically, the situation is further exacerbated by the nature of hostage events as real-life, real-time dramas. Whereas in the case of other terrorist tactics, such as bombings, the news value of the incident is exhausted almost as soon as it is published, in hostage incidents, the breaking of the news about the event is just the beginning of the build-up of tension which is expected to peak at the time of the deadline declared by the terrorists. Throughout this period, the government is subject to contradicting pressures from a variety of sources.

This sketchy portrayal of hostage situations highlights the essence of terrorist tactics in general, and of hostage taking in particular. Such tactics are not aimed at maximizing physical impact but rather political effect. They are predicated on the drawing of authorities into public, widely exposed confrontations and compelling them to act in publicly unacceptable and indefensible ways. In this regard, hostage taking is uniquely advantageous as it can be effectively used to maneuver authorities into "no win" situations: if they concede in order to save hostages, some will criticize them for lack of resolve; if they assume a steadfast stance and hostages die, others will judge them callous and inhumane.

Hostage situations, then, are inherently imbalanced. Except for very rare cases, such as the dramatic release of hostages at Entebbe and Mogadishu, the government cannot win in a hostage affair. At best it can avoid losses. For a terrorist group, the odds are quite opposite: politically it can hardly lose in such situations; often it gains much. It should be stressed, though, that such an imbalance applies to the calculations of the terrorist *organization* that plans and orders the taking of hostages rather than to those of the actual hostage takers. The latter have potentially much to lose: their own lives.

Hostage incidents can be classified into three major types: kidnapping, hijacking, and barricade-and-hostage events. Although in all three the basic situation is similar insofar as terrorists threaten the lives of hostages unless their demands are met, they also differ in some important respects.

In kidnap cases, the hostages are held in a hideout unknown to the government. Communication between the abductors and the government is usually intermittent and indirect (e.g., via messages to news agencies). As long as the location of the kidnapped person or persons is unknown, a forcible release is impossible. These incidents may therefore last for extended periods – weeks, months, or even years. Typically, as time goes on, public interest in the case declines.

Hijack cases mostly involve the forcible takeover of airplanes, but hijackings of buses, trains, and ships have also occurred. Commercial aircraft hijacking is characterized by three elements: the number of hostages is large; they usually include nationals of several countries; and the hijackers are mobile, being often able to choose a landing site that suits their purpose. When the hijacked vehicle is stationary, and located in a territory hostile to the terrorists, the case is essentially a barricade-and-hostage incident. Due to the difficult physical conditions aboard a seized aircraft, these incidents do not last more than a few days.

In barricade-and-hostage events terrorists typically barricade themselves, with their hostages, in a building. Such events constitute a most blatant challenge to authorities as terrorists often stage them, on purpose, in their adversary government's territory. Since the terrorists' location is known and accessible to security forces, the terrorists are declaredly willing to sacrifice themselves if the government opts for a forceful solution. Although these incidents may in principle last indefinitely, they usually come to an end within hours or days. It seems that the political and psychological pressures on the government and the stress of physical danger and uncertainty impinging on the terrorists usually bring about a speedy conclusion. Because the situation is stationary and the location known, barricade-and-hostage incidents gain, at least in democracies, extensive, live media coverage and attract worldwide attention.

The Response: Strategy and Tactics

Strategy: The "Policy Debate"

The response to and handling of hostage situations must be considered, as already pointed out, on two levels: the strategic and the tactical. The former, to which we now address ourselves, concerns the policy that governments should adopt vis-à-vis hostage taking in order to minimize their incidence.

The different views on the policy question are presented in the literature as the "policy debate" (Friedland, 1983; Mickolus, 1976). At the core of this debate are two basic response patterns which govern governments' handling of hostage incidents. One of these patterns is best represented by the American "no concessions" policy which has been repeatedly stated by Unites States officials since 1972. For example, the director of the State Department's Office for Combating Terrorism declared: "We firmly believe that terrorists should be denied benefits from acts such as hostage holding or kidnapping; thus the US Government does not make concessions to blackmail. We will not pay ransom or release prisoners in response to such demands" (Sayre, 1982).

The other approach to hostage events has been termed the "flexible response" (Mickolus, 1976). A leading proponent, in theory and practice, of this approach has described it as follows: "Mixed strategies (delay, negotiation, promises, firmness, consistency, force) used flexibly in different, changing situations and not chained to any preconceived political or other biases produce the best results. I do not advocate softness: To yield under any circumstances is just as unprofitable and futile as to decide in advance never to yield" (Hacker, 1976, p. 228).

The two approaches clearly differ in their underlying assumptions. Advocates of "no concessions" maintain that conceding to terrorists' blackmail amounts to reinforcing their behavior and is thus bound to make it more likely to recur (Friedland, 1983). Proponents of the "flexible response" disagree. For instance, Hacker (1976) claims that "all experience ... proved that terrorist acts, handled nonviolently, are much less likely to be repeated than those settled by violence" (p. 228). Evans (1979) argues from a somewhat different angle that since terrorists' main objective in hostage incidents is publicity, which they get regardless of government policy, practically every hostage case is automatically rewarded from the terrorists' point of view. Therefore, government willingness to sacrifice hostages does not serve its purpose.

One obvious way to attempt a resolution of the "policy debate" is the statistical analysis of the evidence accumulated to date. Unfortunately, the empirical evidence supports neither the "no concessions" nor the "flexible response" policy. Aston (1984) conducted an extensive study of political hostage taking in Europe from 1970 to 1982. He concluded his study with the assertion that "there is ... no clear evidence in Western Europe to suggest that one form of policy has a greater deterrent effect than any other. A deterrent is only effective if the terrorists allow themselves to be deterred and the extent of such deterrence is a matter of speculation" (p. 18).

This ambiguity suggests that the assumptions underlying the two policies may be overly simplistic and that the analysis of the response to hostage taking cannot be based on a simple model of deterrence. We submit, in other words, that social scientists should undertake the development of a more systematic and comprehensive model that specifies the conditions under which a steadfast refusal to concede to hostage takers' demands will lower the recurrence of such incidents and the conditions under which such a policy is likely to fail. Inasmuch as political terrorism is essentially a form of psychological warfare, much can be gained from the involvement of psychologists and, particularly, of social psychologists. Specifically, psychologists could make a significant contribution by systematically investigating areas such as the motivations that shape terrorist action, group dynamics within terrorist organizations, and the decision-making processes in such organizations.

To illustrate the need for a more comprehensive approach it may be pointed out that proponents of the "no concessions" policy and those that advocate a "flexible response" have exclusively addressed themselves to the effects of policy on the decision-making of terrorist organizations. In contrast, a comprehensive model that examines the inner structure and dynamics of terrorist organizations will necessarily distinguish between the motivations and decisions of the "organization – its planners and leaders – and those of the individual members who have to carry out the organization's plans.

As already argued, a terrorist organization can hardly lose in a hostage incident. Yet the actual perpetrators put in jeopardy their own lives. Unless one assumes that the perpetrators are suicidal, the fear of being killed, wounded, or captured may be regarded as a major factor influencing hostage takers' behavior. It is conceivable, therefore, that a hard-line "no concessions" policy might effectively deter individual hostage takers. However, to achieve such effectiveness the emphasis should be placed on deterrence through punishment rather than on the mere withholding of rewards. In other words, the hard-line policy should be reformulated as "punishment for perpetrators" instead of "no concessions."

A diametrically opposed effect may be expected, however, when the reaction of a terrorist organization is considered. It may be conjectured that the organization, facing a hard-line policy, would find it particularly challenging to put it to a test; not only to demonstrate its seriousness, but also because the breaking of a declared policy is particularly damaging to the government and correspondingly rewarding to the organization. One approach that a terrorist organization may adopt to achieve this result consists of maximizing the discrepancy between the value of their pawn and the magnitude of their demands. Thus, if the terrorists manage to seize a large number of particularly sensitive hostages (e. g., children or foreign diplomats) and ask little for their release (say, the publication of a communiqué and safe conduct from the country), any government would find it very difficult to adhere to its steadfast policy. Another possible result of a hard-line policy is a counter-hardening of terrorists' conduct in hostage situations. Having decided to challenge a government's unyielding position, terrorists would try to increase their chance of success by maximizing pressure on authorities. To this effect they are likely to present shorter deadlines, resort to demonstrative killing of hostages, refuse to free wounded or sick hostages, and use frequent interim ultimata to enhance their control over the situation.

This illustration demonstrates the complexity of the strategic facet of the response to hostage taking. The complexity largely stems from the need to address both individual and group processes, and the possibility that success in affecting the individuals in a desired way will produce a diametrically opposite, undesirable effect on the group. Hence, to reiterate, the "policy debate" cannot be settled unless a more comprehensive model of the deterrence of hostage taking is developed.

Tactics: Negotiating with Hostage Takers

Out of recent experience with hostage incidents two general approaches to their resolution have evolved: forceful action and negotiation. The first is of little interest for the present discussion except insofar as its feasibility may affect the likelihood of a negotiated resolution being sought. The second approach poses a challenge to students of bargaining and negotiation: Can bargaining theory be applied to the resolution of hostage incidents?

This query cannot be easily answered since, despite a large number of systematic analyses of the bargaining process (Bacharach & Lawler, 1981; Druckman, 1977; Fisher & Uri, 1981; Morley & Stephenson, 1977; Pruitt, 1981; Raiffa, 1982; Rubin & Brown, 1975; Zartman, 1978), a general theory of bargaining has yet to be developed (cf. Rubin, 1983). Lacking a general theory, we reviewed the bargaining literature, written by social psychologists and other social scientists, in an attempt to identify prerequisites for the effective application of bargaining as a mode of conflict resolution. This review by no means comprises an exhaustive model of bargaining effectiveness. It addresses, however, a number of themes that suffice to evaluate the applicability of bargaining to hostage incidents. These themes are:

1. The core of conflict: the nature of the contested issues.
2. Rationality, credibility, and trust.
3. Bargaining dilemmas.
4. The need to impress others.
5. Interpersonal sensitivity.
6. Commitments to intransigence.

The Core of Conflict: The Nature of the Contested Issues

At the outset of this review, it is important to recognize that not every problem is negotiable and not every contested issue can be settled via bargaining. As proposed by Rubin,

deeply cherished beliefs and values are simply not negotiable: there is no give here, no possibility for concession making. Either we believe in God, capital punishment, and a woman's right to have an abortion, or we do not. These views may change, but they are not negotiable. You are not likely to modify your outlook if I agree to change my own. (1983, pp. 135–136)

Bargaining is an interactive process, applicable to the resolution of conflict among parties that are dependent on each other for the achievement of their goals. Clearly, conflicting parties are unlikely to engage in bargaining unless they believe that they have a common problem to solve; that is, if they believe that alternative, unilateral acts will provide them with better outcomes. Thus, bargaining requires that there be a *bargaining range,* a set of potential settlements that are preferred by all parties to the outcomes they could obtain without bargaining, or to those they would obtain if bargaining were attempted and failed (cf. Schelling, 1960).

The existence of a bargaining range depends on two factors: the parties' demand levels and the nature of issues at stake. The first factor needs little elaboration. Clearly, if one party's minimal demands fall short of the maximum that the other is willing to concede, there is little room for negotiation. The second factor is more central to our discussion. A bargaining range can only exist when the contested issues or commodities are divisible or exchangeable. Thus bargaining is usually applicable to the division or exchange of tangible or quantifiable assets. Conversely, it is a poor or worthless mode of conflict resolution when the core of conflict consists of intangible, indivisible or inexchangeable isses, such as the beliefs and principles exemplified in Rubin's illustration.

Given this characterization of negotiable issues, a key question concerning the applicability of bargaining and negotiation can now be stated: Do hostage incidents have a bargaining range?

The answer is complex as it depends on the weight given by the parties to material as opposed to political or to tangible versus intangible aspects of the hostage incident. When hostage takers are primarily concerned with the maximization of tangible, material gains such as ransom money or the release of jailed comrades and the target government's main or sole concern is the safe release of the hostages, a bargaining range may be found. Under such circumstances, each party is in full control of the assets desired by the other and each may perceive in the situation a range of potential settlements that are preferable to any outcome it could secure without negotiating.

These assumptions about the existence of a bargaining range may prove to be quite unrealistic in the context of politically motivated hostage incidents. Cases where the sole concern of political terrorists is the maximization of material gains are rare. As already argued, hostage tactics are typically employed to inflict political damage on the target government, to maneuver it into a "no win" situation and to discredit it in the eyes of its consittuents. Likewise, from a target government's perspective, the material consequences of a hostage incident often have a secondary importance. The payment of ransom money is unlikely to upset a country's economy and the release of several jailed terrorists is hardly a threat to national security. A target government is usually more concerned with the political ramifications of its actions; the effects of such actions on the future incidence of hostage taking and their judgment in the court of public opinion. We suggest, then, that politically motivated hostage takers and target governments usually compete for intangible assets: credibility, reputation, appearances, and the praise of relevant constituencies. Such assets are gained or lost in the arena of public opinion, and the public characteristically tends to judge the performance of terrorists and authorities in absolute, categorical terms rather than in graduated, continuous values. Thus, the contested issues in the confrontation between politically motivated hostage takers and governments are not only intangible but also indivisible. Under such circumstances, the confrontation is likely to be devoid of a bargaining range.

The likelihood of identifying a bargaining range in politically motivated hostage incidents is additionally lowered by the imbalance inherent in such situations. The terrorists, as argued, can hardly lose while the target government can rarely win. Hence, hostage situations often lack the mutual dependence for the achievement of outcomes which defines the bargaining range and constitutes a primary motivator for the conduct of genuine negotiation.

Rationality, Credibility, and Trust

Bargaining effectiveness depends on the existence of certain interpersonal perceptions and attitudes. Most notable among these are interpersonal trust, the credibility of the adversary's commitments, and assumptions about the adversary's rationality.

A joint problem-solving approach, which is most conducive to the resolution of conflict, is unlikely to be adopted unless the conflicting parties show at least a modicum of interpersonal trust. Here, the term "trust" carries two meanings. First, it implies a belief in the truthfulness of the adversary's statements. Second, it denotes the expectation that the adversary is aware of and sufficiently concerned about one's own interest, and is therefore ready to engage in joint problem-solving (cf. Pruitt, 1983). Empirical evidence that trust, especially in the second meaning of the term, encourages a problem-solving orientation was found by a number of researchers (e.g., Kimmel, Pruitt, Magenau, Konar-Goldband, & Carnevale, 1980).

Effective bargaining also requires that the adversary be perceived as rational. This specifically means the assumption that the adversary's objectives, aspirations, and demand levels are not subject to change during the bargaining process (Baldwin, 1976). Thus, for example, it is doubtful that bargaining could be effectively conducted and concluded if in response to one party's conciliatory move the other presented new, exorbitant demands.

Lastly, many of the tactics used by bargainers are essentially conditional commitments, different forms of threats and promises (Schelling, 1960). To be effective in bringing about the settlement of conflict, such commitments must be credible; that is, they must be perceived as truly and fully conditional. Conversely, bargaining can rarely progress to a favorable conclusion if one party doubts the conditionality of the other's commitments. Baldwin (1976) illustrated this point with the example of a sadist who "may have no difficulty convincing others of his willingness to carry out his threat, but he may have great difficulty in assuring others that he will refrain from carrying it out if his demands are met" (p. 414).

These conditions for effective bargaining cast some doubt on its applicability to the resolution of hostage incidents. It is hardly necessary to assert that the conditions under which such bargaining has to take place do not promote trust. Moreover, authorities entrusted with the conduct of such negotiations may have reasons to doubt the rationality of the hostage takers or to assume that the tremendous pressure or fatigue impinging on the hostage takers might temporarily impair the rationality of their decisions and actions (cf. Baldwin, 1976). Lastly, the parties to a hostage incident, particularly the hostage takers, may face grave difficulties in proving the conditionality of their commitments. Schelling provided an illuminating example of this difficulty: "Both the kidnapper who would like to release his prisoner, and the prisoner, may search desperately for a way to commit the latter against informing on his captor, without finding one" (1960, p. 43).

Bargaining Dilemmas

The success of bargaining depends to a significant degree on the bargainers' ability to solve a number of dilemmas (Rubin, 1983). First, as various researchers have indicated (Deutsch, 1982; Kelley, 1966; Pruitt, 1981), bargainers must contend with the self-contradictory, mixed-motive nature of the bargaining situation: each is motivated to compete in order to gain the lion's share, but both must cooperate so as to prevent mutual loss.

Second, each bargainer has to strike a delicate balance between absolute honesty and total misrepresentation (Kelley, 1966). The former subjects one to exploitation by the adversary, while misrepresentation and excessive withholding of information engender distrust.

Third, the bargainer must chart the optimal course between the pulls of short-term and long-term outcomes. Often, in order to assure mutual trust, satisfaction, and long-term gains, a negotiator must sacrifice and compromise immediate outcomes (see, e.g., Cross and Guyer, 1980; Platt, 1973).

These dilemmas are extremely difficult to resolve in the context of hostage situations. The difficulty is most salient with respect to the third, as governments faced with hostage incidents typically pursue two highly incompatible goals: the immediate goal of safely releasing the hostages and the long-term goal of deterring future hostage abductions. Thus, the type of balancing that a bargainer faced with, say, a commercial exchange can make ("I'll forego some profit now to assure a certain level of gain in the long haul") cannot be easily applied to hostage incidents. The decision, "I'll sacrifice a few hostages now ..." is too awesome even to contemplate, and is certainly inconsistent with democratic ethics that prohibit the sacrifice of individuals for a greater common good.

The Need to Impress Others

Brown (1968, 1970) has demonstrated the consequences of negotiators' efforts to maintain "face" and an appearance of strength. The resolution of conflict can be considerably hindered when the parties assign a high importance to the impressions they make on their adversaries and constituencies. As was the case with Brown's experimental subjects, negotiators may at times go to the lengths of accepting financial or other material losses in order to maintain or restore their reputation.

If the need to maintain face can at times become an important factor in negotiations concerning tangible issues, it would without exception play a most detrimental role in hostage incidents. These, after all, are initiated by terrorists in order to tarnish the reputation and credibility of target governments, and their outcomes, as argued, are measured in terms of impressions made on relevant publics. Moreover, in hostage situations it is rarely possible to apply procedures designed to attenuate the detrimental effects of face-saving motivations. For instance, attempts to move negotiations out of the limelight and conduct them in secrecy are usually unrealistic, considering the active involvement of the news media in hostage situations (Rubin & Friedland, 1986). A more promising possibility is to rely on the face-saving potential of third party mediation (cf. Meeker & Shure, 1969; Podell & Knapp,1969; Pruitt & Johnson, 1970). Yet governments are often reluctant to enlist neutral intermediaries since such a move might be perceived as a sign of helplessness and an admission of defeat. In addition, third party intervention might commit them to concessions they would not otherwise make and it might interfere with or prevent forceful action.

Interpersonal Sensitivity

Sensitivity to the needs, desires, and motivations of the adversary are important for the effective conduct of negotiations. This proposition is qualified by findings showing that too high a level of sensitivity might induce excessive reactivity to the actions of the opponent and thereby enhance the risk of less than optimal settlements (Rubin & Brown, 1975; Swap & Rubin, 1983; Kelley & Schenitzki, 1972). Yet a certain degree of sensitivity is nevertheless needed in order to anticipate the opponent's response to one's moves and to decipher the true meaning behind the opponent's positions and tactics.

The physical conditions under which the dialogue and exchange between hostage takers and authorities typically takes place often hamper sound judgment of the adversary's motivations and intentions. This is most obviously the case in kidnappings and hijackings, where communication between the abductors and authorities is indirect and intermittent (e.g., via news agencies or through messages transmitted by the pilot of a seized airliner). These situations, then, preclude a face-to-face, flowing communication, without which a reasonably valid assessment of the adversary is hardly possible. Yet even in barricade-and-hostage situations, where, technically, more direct and continuous communication can be held, such assessment is difficult. For one thing, the parties can (and hostage takers often do) deliberately disrupt communication. Second, it is not always clear whether each party's spokesperson is empowered to make decisions or is merely a conduit of messages. Hence, judgments based on the spokesperson's behavior and apparent state of mind can lead to erroneous conclusions.

Additional difficulty in the judgment and assessment of the adversary stems from the unique "dramaturgical" qualities of hostage incidents. These are likened by Friedland and Rubin (unpublished observations) to a drama enacted on a multisided stage, each side facing a different audience, each audience being unaware of the others. Thus, messages exchanged in the course of a hostage incident may often be complex and ambiguous, contain both explicit and hidden meanings, and therefore difficult to interpret and decipher.

Commitment to Intransigence

The negotiated resolution of conflict is usually brought about by the application of commitment tactics. These are designed to compel the adversary to yield by convincing him or her that one will not go back on a commitment to a certain position. Without such tactics, the bargaining process could turn into a highly inefficient, lengthy sequence of offers and counteroffers that does not reach a resting point (cf. Schelling, 1960). Commitment tactics, however, are a double-edged sword. If the adversary does not yield, the committed party is left with the painful choice between having to undo the commitment, lose credibility and subject itself to subsequent exploitation, or, alternatively, effect a stalemate. Hence, though the use of commitment tactics can hardly be avoided, they should be used with extreme caution.

Commitment tactics can be applied within a tolerable margin of risk if two conditions are met. The first condition quite obviously requires that the commitment be credible and made to be perceived as truly binding. Second, commitments should only be made to potential settlements that are contained in the bargaining range. These, by definition, are preferred by both parties to a stalemate or to the discontinuation of negotiations. Thus, if one party convincingly commits itself to such a settlement, the other is left with no alternative but to yield. Conversely, if a party commits itself to a settlement that is outside the bargaining range, the other has no incentive to yield and may in fact respond with a countercommitment (cf. Friedland, 1983). In this event bargaining will grind to a standstill and, in extreme cases, the dynamics of brinkmanship will take over.

The potential risks associated with commitment tactics are inescapable in hostage situations. First, the involved parties may find great difficulty in making their commitments credible. As argued above, the hostage takers will find it easy to convince authorities of their determination to hurt the hostages if their demands are not met, but they may find it difficult to assure authorities that the hostages would come to no harm if their demands are met. Second, as also already argued, hostage incidents have an extremely narrow bargaining range. Hence, commitments, rather than effecting agreements, are likely to turn hostage incidents into highly volatile situations.

The high risk associated with the use of commitment tactics in hostage situations might lead one to the conclusion that such tactics should be avoided altogether. This is hardly possible, however, as the very initiation of a hostage incident requires a commitment. That is, terrorists would make themselves a laughing-stock if they threatened: "Release our jailed comrades, otherwise we'll hijack a plane!" They start by hijacking the plane, and leave authorities the task of undoing the commitment.

Particular prerequisites for effective bargaining and the likelihood of satisfying them in hostage incidents have been reviewed, it is now possible to consider the general question posed at the outset: Can bargaining be applied to the resolution of hostage incidents?

Some of the potential obstacles to the effective use of bargaining in hostage incidents appear insurmountable. These include lack of trust, low credibility and interpersonal sensitivity, and doubts about the rationality of the adversary. Given the antecedents and nature of conflict between hostage takers and authorities, as well as the conditions prevailing in hostage incidents, it is difficult to conceive of circumstances that will allow the involved parties to regard their opponents as trustworthy, credible, and sufficiently rational.

Although these impediments to the application of bargaining are by no means trivial, they do not completely rule out a negotiated solution. The feasibility of bargaining more importantly depends on hostage takers' and authorities' ability to identify an integrative potential or, in different terms, on the existence of a sufficiently wide bargaining range. This depends, in turn, on the basic orientation of the involved parties and on their ability and willingness to contain the public-directed effects of their actions.

The first of these two conditions refers to the relative weight given by both hostage takers and authorities to concrete, tangible issues compared with intangible ones. Thus, if hostage takers apply themselves to the receipt of material ranson, ignoring publicity and the desire to inflict political damage on the target government, and the latter addresses itself to the release of hostages, putting aside political ramifications and the establishment of precedent, a bargaining range can often be established. Such an orientation can only be assumed, however, under a condition of low accountability, where the need to impress publics and constituents is minimal. Hence, the second condition proposed above: that the feasibility of applying bargaining to the resolution of hostage incidents importantly depends on the practicality of concealing the unfolding of such incidents from the public view.

Are these two conditions likely to be met in hostage situations? Our analysis of terrorist strategy and tactics indicates that the likelihood is rather low. The primary objectives of political terrorists are political rather than material. Their tactics, as previously argued, are predicated on the drawing of authorities into widely exposed confrontations and forcing them to act in ways unacceptable to the public. Hence, an issue-oriented approach that gives precedence to the potential material outcomes of a hostage incident contradicts the very essence of political terrorism. Political terrorists will accordingly make every possible effort to enhance the political significance and public impact of hostage incidents. In turn, target governments, faced with a continuous and recurring political challenge, have no alternative to responding according to largely political considerations.

The importance accorded by parties to a hostage incident to the political significance of their actions augments the weight of indivisible intangibles at the core of conflict. These tend to obfuscate any integrative potential that might exist in such situations, making bargaining and negotiation highly unlikely. Therefore, the probable outcomes of such situations are victory to one party or loss to both. In more operational terms, the likely outcomes are either the capitulation of one party or violent action. Rarely will a hostage incident be concluded with a negotiated "50% solution" such as is common in other types of conflict. Paul Wilkinson (1981) was therefore right in concluding that the term "hostage negotiations" is a misnomer.

The preceding propositions suggest that the study and analysis of hostage incidents will achieve little if they remain confined to the context of negotiation theory. What is needed is a conceptual reframing of such incidents and a clearer characterization of the processes that shape them. If hostage "negotiations" is a misnomer, how should one label the confrontation and exchange between hostage takers and authorities?

An answer to this query can be found by applying Pruitt and Rubin's (1986) model of strategic choice in conflict. This model singles out low interpersonal trust, a refusal to accept the legitimacy of the adversary's concerns, and the lack of integrative potential as conditions that drive conflicting parties away from a joint problem-solving orientation, which is the heart of the bargaining process, toward the adoption of contentious strategies. Thus, the problem of hostage takers and authorities, as they see it, is not the just division of the pie; rather, each party undertakes the task of compelling the other to give up and yield its slice of the pie. Under these circumstances, most hostage incidents are likely to degenerate into potentially volatile tests of brinkmanship.

Brinkmanship differs from bargaining in the nature of the commitments that the parties employ to bring conflict to a conclusion. Bargaining, as argued by Schelling (1960), reaches a settlement when one party convincingly commits itself to a mutually satisfying solution, i. e., a solution which is contained in the bargaining range. Brinkmanship, on the other hand, is employed in conflicts that lack a bargaining range. Hence, the essence of brinkmanship is a strong and seemingly irrevocable commitment to a mutually *destructive* course of action which burdens the adversary with the responsibility for averting mutual disaster. The upper hand in a contest of brinkmanship is gained by the party which is determined enough, desperate enough, or crazy enough to make a truly binding commitment to mutual damage.

The characterization of hostage incidents as contests of brinkmanship suggests that their understanding requires that they be examined from a wide psychological perspective. Bargaining models that are largely addressed to issues and tactics are insufficient, for in brinkmanship the personalities and motivations of the parties become the decisive factors. None of the existing bargaining models can predict the circumstances under which hostage takers will take the life of a hostage or the behavior of a government representative faced with awesome, split-second decisions. It appears then that students of personality and clinical psychologists have much to contribute to the understanding of hostage incidents.

Contests of brinkmanship subject the contestants to extreme stress. In hostage situations, hostage takers often put their lives on the line and authorities are called to determine the fate of the hostages. Hence, an additional significant contribution can be made by experts on behavior under stress and, particularly, on decision making under Stress.

Lastly, one should not lose sight of the fact that hostage incidents are real-life dramas, enacted in front of an audience, and that the involved parties behave according to assumptions about the effects of their actions on relevant publics and constituents. Therefore, a systematic study of these assumptions and their validity, of the attitudinal impact of hostage incidents on the public and, conversely, of the effects of public opinion on both authorities and terrorists may shed light on the dynamics and unfolding of hostage incidents.

Summary

In the preceding pages we have attempted to describe the main features of political hostage taking and the problems inherent in the design of effective response to hostage tactics. Political hostage taking, unlike that which is motivated by criminal or mercenary reasons, should not be regarded as a mere act of extortion. For the politically motivated hostage taker, the attainment of concrete, tangible outcomes such as ransom money or the release of jailed comrades is secondary. Political effects and attitudinal impact on relevant publics are paramount and these, as shown, are only marginally related to the magnitude of target government concessions.

The outcomes sought by political terrorists confront target governments with difficulties and dilemmas concerning both policies and tactics. Regarding the former, policy makers have to choose between the "flexible response" and "no concessions" policies. The choice is obviously difficult and the empirical evidence accumulated to date on the effects of the two policies provides little guidance. A systematic analysis by students of social influence and deterrence is thus sorely needed.

On the tactical level, target governments usually waver between two incompatible goals: securing the release of hostages and earning a reputation for firmness that will deter future hostage taking. The latter goal adds to the weight of intangible issues at the core of conflict and severely constricts the bargaining range. Under such circumstances, the direct application of bargaining know-how and tactics to the resolution of hostage incidents may prove ineffective or counterproductive. This does not imply, however, that students of bargaining should be excluded from the analysis of hostage situations. It takes bargaining know-how to know why bargaining can rarely be applied to the resolution of hostage incidents. Thus, though bargaining theory does not offer a winning strategy for hostage situations, it may at least help avoid losing strategies.

Hostage incidents were shown to be highly complex and risky situations, where each party must withstand a multitude of conflicting pressures and each can only hope to prevail by eroding the resolve and determination of the other. Psychology can doubtlessly make a highly significant contribution to both the analysis and management of such incidents. However, to realise this potential contribution, three conditions have to be met. First, it must be recognized that hostage incidents are extreme and explosive situations. Psychologists, who typically address themselves to the broadest commonalities of human behavior, should therefore be extremely cautious in applying their knowledge to the investigation and management of hostage situations. Second, psychologists' involvement is bound to prove fruitless if they adopt a piecemeal, narrow disciplinary approach. The complexity of hostage situations requires that they be examined with a wide range of conceptual and analytic tools. In other words, knowledge from many branches of psychology must be simultaneously applied. Third, hostage incidents must be examined in the political and social context in which they occur. These incidents resemble in many ways theatrical productions. But they are productions in which the audience plays an active and critically important role. Hence, analyses of hostage incidents are bound to remain incomplete without a thorough consideration of the intricate relationship between the main parties, on the one hand, and publics and constituents on the other.

References

Aston, J.Z. (1984). Political hostage taking in Western Europe. *Conflict Studies, 157*, 1–21.
Bacharach, S.B., & Lawler, E.J. (1981). *Bargaining: Power, tactics and outcomes*. San Francisco: Jossey-Bass.
Baldwin, D.A. (1976). Bargaining with airline hijackers. In I.W.Zartman (Ed.) *The 50% solution*. New York: Doubleday.
Brown, B.R. (1968). The effects of need to maintain face on interpersonal bargaining. *Journal of Experimental Social Psychology, 4*, 107–122.

Brown, B. R. (1970). Face saving following experimentally induced embarrassment. *Journal of Experimental Social Psychology, 6,* 255–271.

Cross, J. G., & Guyer, M. J. (1980). *Social traps.* Ann Arbor: University of Michigan Press.

Deutsch, M. (1982). *The resolution of conflict.* New Haven: Yale University Press.

Druckman, D. (1977). *Negotiations: Social psychological perspectives.* Beverly Hills: Sage.

Evans, E. (1979). *Calling a truce to terror.* Westport: Greenwood.

Fisher, R., & Uri, W. (1981). *Getting to yes: Negotiating agreement without giving in.* Boston! Houghton Mifflin.

Friedland, N. (1983). Hostage negotiations: Dilemmas about policy. In L. Z. Freedman & Y. Alexander (Eds.), *Perspectives on terrorism.* Wilmington: Scholarly Resources.

Friedland, N. (1983). Weakness as strength: The use and misuse of a "my hands are tied" ploy in bargaining. *Journal of Applied Social Psychology, 13,* 422–426.

Hacker, F. J. (1976). *Crusaders, criminals, crazies.* New York: Norton.

Kelley, H. H. (1966). A classroom study of the dilemmas in interpersonal negotiations. In K. Archibald (Ed.), *Strategic interaction and conflict.* Berkeley: Institute of International Studies.

Kelley, H. H., & Schenitzki, D. P. (1972). Bargaining. In C. G. McClintock (Ed.), *Experimental social psychology.* New York: Holt.

Kimmel, D., Pruitt, D. G., Magenau, J. M., Konar-Goldband, E., & Carnevale, P. J. D. (1980). Effects of trust aspiration and gender on negotiation tactics. *Journal of Personality and Social Psychology, 38,* 9–23.

Meeker, R. J., & Shure, G. H. (1969). Pacifist bargaining tactics. *Journal of Conflict Resolution, 13,* 487–493.

Mickolus, E. F. (1976). Negotiations for hostages: A policy dilemma. *Orbis, 19,* 1309–1326.

Morley, I. E., & Stephenson, G. M. (1977). *The social psychology of bargaining.* London: Allen & Unwin.

Platt, J. (1973). Social traps. *American Psychologist, 28,* 641–651.

Podell, J. E., & Knapp, W. M. (1969). The effect of mediation on the perceived firmness of the opponent. *Journal of Conflict Resolution, 13,* 511–520.

Pruitt, D. G. (1981). *Negotiation behavior.* New York: Academic.

Pruitt, D. G. (1983). Strategic choice in negotiation. *American Behavioral Scientist, 27,* 167–194.

Pruitt, D. G., & Johnson, D. F. (1970). Mediation as an aid to face saving in negotiation. *Journal of Personality and Social Psychology, 14,* 239–246.

Pruitt, D. G., & Rubin, J. Z. (1986). *Social conflict: Escalation. stalemate, and settlement.* New York: Random House.

Raiffa, H. (1982). *The art and science of negotiation.* Cambridge, MA: Harvard University Press.

Rubin, J. Z. (1983). Negotiation: An introduction to some issues and themes. *American Behavioral Scientist, 27,* 135–148.

Rubin, J. Z., & Brown, B. R. (1975). *The social psychology of bargaining and negotiation.* New York: Academic.

Rubin, J. Z., & Friedland, N. (1986). Negotiating with terrorists. *Psychology Today, 20,* 18–28.

Sayre, R. M. (1982). Combatting terrorism: American policy and organization. In United States Department of State, Bureau of Public Affairs, *Combatting Terrorism.* Washington, DC: US Government Printing Office.

Schelling, T. C. (1960). *The strategy of conflict.* Cambridge, MA: Harvard University Press.

Swap, W. C., & Rubin, J. Z. (1983). Measurement of interpersonal orientation. *Journal of Personality and Social Psychology, 44,* 208–219.

Wilkinson, P. (1981). Admissibility of negotiations between organs of the democratic state and terrorists. In *Conference on the defense of democracy against terrorism in Europe,* (Council of Europe Compendium of Documents). Strasbourg, November 1980.

Zartman, I. W. (Ed.). (1978). *The negotiation process: Theories and applications.* Beverly Hills: Sage.

Chapter 9

Intergroup Contact, Cultural Information, and Change in Ethnic Attitudes

Rachel Ben-Ari and Yehuda Amir

The problem of intergroup conflict has been a major concern for numerous societies and countries in the world. Intergroup tensions exist between blacks and whites in the USA, between the white and colored populations in Britain, between the native population and immigrant workers in the Federal Republic of Germany, and in many other regions of the world where intergroup prejudice and hostility culminate in violence and bloodshed.

According to Secord and Backman (1974), the nature of the relations between groups determines the nature of their mutual attitudes. In the case of positive relations, positive attitudes and perceptions will develop, but in the case of a conflict, discrimination and prejudice will follow. Indeed, it has been shown that conflict between groups usually causes the development of hostility, prejudice, and stereotypes (Hofman, 1977; Rabbie & Horwitz, 1969; Sherif, Harvey, White, Hood & Sherif, 1961; Sinha & Upadhyaya, 1960). These findings support Campbell's "realistic conflict theory" (1965) according to which prejudice, discrimination, and the rejection of people from a "different group" stem from a real conflict between them. One may conjecture, therefore, that when a conflict is resolved, its by-products, including negative attitudes and perceptions which have influenced intergroup relations, may also disappear. In reality, however, this is not as simple as it sounds. First, there are conflicts which are not or cannot be resolved, and one has to learn to live with them while coexisting with the other group. For example, Arabs and Jews in Israel have to function together even if no solution is found for the political conflict and/or if the differences between them do not change. Moreover, even when the conflict is terminated, some of its by-products or consequences may continue to exist and affect the groups' behavior. Ethnic attitudes and stereotypes seem to reinforce themselves regardless of the real existence of the conflict. Thus, in addition to the search for the resolution of the conflict which is generally in the macro level (e.g., political, economic) spheres, techniques should be developed and implemented at the micro level to deal with products of the conflict, such as the mutual attitudes and perceptions of the people involved in it.

Two approaches are generally suggested to deal with the outcomes of intergroup conflict: the "contact approach" based on physical contact between
members of the groups in conflict, and the "information approach" focused on
the information available to the members of one group about the other one. In
this chapter we shall try to evaluate the effectiveness of combining these two
approaches for changing interethnic attitudes.

First, intergroup contact will be presented as a way for changing intergroup
relations and attitudes. There are, however, certain cognitive aspects which may
limit its effectiveness in producing such a change. Therefore, the notion will be
advanced that it is possible to overcome these limitations by constructing the
contact situation according to certain principles and by cognitively preparing
the individuals involved in the contact situation. Following these theoretical
considerations, a study will be reported which has combined these two approaches and evaluated this integrative attempt in tourism, specifically regarding visits of Israelis to Egypt.

Contact – A Way to Change Ethnic Attitudes

Back in the 1940s and early 1950s, it was generally believed that intergroup
contact would inevitably improve the mutual attitudes and relations of the interacting members. It was assumed that mere contact among individuals from
diverse groups creates an opportunity for mutual acquaintance, enhances understanding and acceptance among the interacting group members, and consequently reduces intergroup prejudice, conflict, and tension. This belief has fostered national policy decisions in the areas of housing, work, and education, as
well as various international programs of student exchanges, professional conferences, sport, etc. The beliefs in the efficacy of contact are based, in part, on
the empirical findings summarized and reviewed by Allport (1954), Amir (1969,
1976), Cook (1962), and others. These reviewers conclude that contact often
changes attitudes and relations between diverse ethnic groups. The importance
of contact was heightened by recognition that other approaches to intergroup
relations have not proven successful (Ashmore, 1970).

The theoretical rationale behind the contact hypothesis is often based on
cognitive considerations. It is generally assumed that the development of negative stereotypes and attitudes stems from the absence of sufficient information
and/or the existence of erroneous information held by one group about the
other one. Contact situations provide new information and the opportunity for
clarification and for relearning. As individuals discover that "others" are more
similar to themselves than was assumed (Rokeach, 1960) or even hold similar
attitudes (Byrne, 1969; Newcomb, 1961), they tend to discard negative attitudes
or to develop positive ones towards the "others."

Limitations of the Contact Approach

In this light, of course, successful contact requires that interacting individuals are receptive to the new information. However, the literature suggests that several processes operate during contact which hinder the process of relearning. One process is social categorization (Tajfel, 1961), which strengthens the individual's tendency to accentuate intracategory similarity and intercategory differences. This simplifies the cognitive organization of the complex network of social groups encountered by the individual and eases social judgments. In such a case, the accentuation preserves different value systems for the different social groups. Taylor, Fiske, Etcoff, and Ruderman (1978) suggested that as a result of social categorization, intragroup differences are minimized, whereas intergroup differences are maximized. In addition, the individual tends to perceive the members of his own group in a more positive way than the members of the other group.

A second barrier to contact effects, according to theories of social identity or social comparison, is the tendency to prefer one's own group characteristics, even in the absence of conflict or explicit competition with others. This tendency stems from the need to attain or preserve a positive social identity for the group (Tajfel, 1981). It can be assumed, then, that an individual will exhibit various forms of resistance to any new information which can disrupt the existing psychological balance.

Dynamic features of stereotypes may also hinder acquisition of new information. Hamilton (1979) argues that stereotypes constitute a structural framework for processing new information and functions as a schema (Kelley, 1972). This schema sensitizes the individual to elements in the environment that are consistent with it and dismisses inconsistent elements. Stereotypes are related to characteristics attributed to in- and outgroups. Information inconsistent with stereotypes can be dismissed by attributing the facts to influences rather than to the group member himself.

In view of these barriers, it seems that the effectiveness of contact depends not only on the kind of information provided in the contact situation, but also on the participant's openness to that information. Contact, therefore, should be regarded as a necessary but not sufficient condition for producing a positive change in ethnic attitudes and relations. In order for contact to be effective, it must take place under conditions of "positive exposure" which circumvent these barriers. Findings that intergroup contact does not always improve group relations and sometimes even increases tension and hostility (Bloom, 1971; Tajfel & Dawson, 1965) bolster the notion that the efficacy of contact depends on the surrounding conditions.

Conditions of Positive Exposure

Conditions of positive exposure are summarized by Amir (1969, 1976) and Cook (1970). They include:

1. Equal-status contact between the members of the interacting groups. Unfortunately, this is generally difficult to achieve in contact situations between majority and minority groups. Still, change may also be produced if important characteristics of the interacting minority members are different from and more positive than the stereotypes held by majority members with regard to these characteristics.
2. Intergroup cooperation in the pursuit of common goals. This kind of situation creates an interdependence between the groups and discourages competition which hinders positive change.
3. Contact of intimate rather than casual nature which allows the interacting members to get to know each other beyond the superficial level.
4. An "authority" and/or social climate approving of and supporting the intergroup contact. Of particular relevance here is the support given to intergroup contact by the community, social institutions, friends, or any "relevant others."

The necessity of positive exposure conditions has been found to hold in many areas of intergroup contact (Amir, 1969, 1976; Miller, 1981; St.John, 1975) including Arab-Jewish relationships in Israel (Amir, 1979; Amir & Ben-Ari, 1985; Amir, Ben-Ari, Bizman, & Rivner, 1980, 1982).

Reviews of the exposure conditions cited by Amir and Cook reveal a focus on structural features of the contact situation and ignore the personal features of the participant, i.e., initial intergroup attitudes, the intensity of his intergroup feelings, and his readiness for intergroup contact. Yet such personal features may determine the individual's openness to accepting and integrating information about the others. Stephan and Stephan (1984) and Landis, Hope, and Day (1984) stress knowledge and acceptance of intergroup differences as prior conditions to interpersonal acceptance. Information about outgroup members is likely to be rejected or assimilated to preexisting negative stereotypes unless alternative knowledge structures are available to process and organize the information effectively. The provision of new knowledge about the outgroup prior to contact may establish such alternative structures.

Providing Information – A Way to Change Ethnic Attitudes

The transfer of new knowledge brings us to the crux of a second approach to improving intergroup relations: the information approach. This approach stresses the supply of information to one group about the other one through mass communication or educational programs. The main assumption here is that ignorance and lack of information comprise the first stage in the development of prejudice, stereotypes, and the consequent tension between groups (Myrdal, 1944; Williams, 1947). Indeed, negative correlations have been found between educational level and the extent of prejudices and discriminatory tendencies toward outgroups (Harding, Proshansky, Kutner, & Chein, 1969; Wagner & Schoenbach, 1984). Furthermore, correlations between ignorance of ethnic outgroups and prejudice also bolster this thesis (Bolton, 1935; Murphy & Likert, 1938; Nettler, 1946).

Programs based on the information approach generally focus on the history of the different groups in the society, highlight their achievement and contributions, and stress the similarity between the groups. Among the evaluated 39 programs in this area which were summarized by Stephan and Stephan (1984), 24 found that educational materials succeeded in reducing prejudice, 14 found no effects, and one even found an increase in prejudice.

Some intervention programs stress group differences. Here misperceptions and real dissimilarities are assumed to be the bases of conflict. According to this view, programs should explain and legitimize the differences between groups rather than ignore them. This tack on information use has generally been applied in programs dealing with cross-cultural differences (Brislin, Cushner, Cherrie, & Yong, 1986; Triandis, 1975).

There are empirical findings to indicate the effectiveness of the information approach (Davis & Fine; 1975; Stephan & Stephan, 1984). On the other hand, others have shown no such effect (Cooper & Dinerman, 1951; Crawford, 1984). One major problem with the information approach is that people who regard the other group negatively often do not wish to be exposed to such a program and, if they cannot avoid it, may distort its message (Berelson & Steiner, 1964).

Combining the Contact and Informational Approaches

As shown above, both approaches have the potential for changing intergroup attitudes but also some limitations to achieving this. We suggested testing the effectiveness of combining both approaches.

Our suggestion was to provide cognitive training (information) before the behavioral experience (contact) in order to optimally prepare the individual to the exposure during the contact experience. Preparation refers here to the modification of the individual's schema about the other group. This will consequently enable the individual to assimilate new information or ensure that the new information provided during the contact falls within the latitude of acceptance rather than within the latitude of rejection, in the terms of Hovland, Harvey, and Sherif (1957).

In order to test the notion about the effectiveness of consolidating the information and contact approaches, one has to search for a real situation in which the two approaches can be utilized. Intergroup contact in a tourist setting seemed to provide such an opportunity. Therefore, we decided to evaluate the contact between Israelis and Egyptians during a tour by Israelis in Egypt.

Contact between Israelis and Egyptians

With the signing of the Egyptian-Israel peace treaty, Israelis and Egyptians are now free to visit a country that was recently enemy territory and meet a nation that has been an object of negative attitudes and hostility. This development provides an interesting field setting for testing the effects of the intergroup contact on the mutual attitudes and relations between the two nations.

What are the characteristics of this setting? Unfortunately, it has a number of features which may lead to category-based social perception. Such categories are more likely to be salient if they are characterized by convergent boundaries (Brewer & Campbell, 1976) in which group identities are based on many different distinctions. "Egyptian" and "Israeli" are social categories that are differentiated by convergent boundaries, including distinctions in terms of their culture, history, religion, nationality, and even physical features. Moreover, the continuous fighting (about 30 years) between the two countries has emphasized the political policies that affect these groups differentially and brings these individuals into the situation as representatives of their respective social categories. Secondly, most of the conditions for "positive exposure", requiring new positive information about the other group in order to facilitate the process of changing attitudes and relationships, are difficult to obtain and, indeed, are not present in the contact between Israelis and Egyptians within a tourism setting. In such a situation, a new information source and psychological preparation are required in order to achieve "positive exposure."

In order to obtain these requirements, an information program was constructed for the (Jewish) Israeli tourists to Egypt. This intervention took into account the cognitive processes that may be present during intergroup contact, e.g., selective perception of the encountered reality (in this present case, emphasizing negative aspects of Egypt), accentuation of intergroup differences, and distortion in the attribution processes.

The intervention program was built with the aim of modifying and moderating these processes and included the following elements:

1. An emphasis on the positive aspects of Egypt and the Egyptians. This is especially important since regular tourist packages emphasize the attractions of ancient Egypt: present-day Egypt is shown only incidentally and what is shown does not represent modern Egypt, but is selected because of its special attractiveness to the tourist. It includes Cairo's "City of the Dead" (a huge slum area built in the area of an old cemetery with a population of 1–2 million), Potter's Village (a large, backward section of Cairo where pottery is produced by ancient and primitive techniques and methods), and downtown Cairo and its market (though picturesque and highly attractive to tourists, these are crowded, dirty, poor, and physically run-down areas). These sights portray Egypt in a biased way, completely overlooking a different Egypt which includes modern dwelling areas – clean, with green open spaces – advanced industry, new, highly developed suburban towns around Cairo, etc. The average visitor to Egypt hardly knows of the existence of

these places. Thus, if one plans to achieve positive attitude changes, it is important to inform the tourist (Israeli or any other) about the positive aspects of Egypt and the Egyptians, thereby giving him or her a more rounded and balanced view of the land and its people.

2. An emphasis on the similarities between the Israeli and the Egyptian. This component was aimed at moderating the process of accentuation of differences between the two peoples and enhancing intergroup attraction.

3. The provision of rational explanations for some of the negative phenomena encountered by the Israeli in Egypt. Israelis tend to attribute such negative phenomena to basic characteristics of the Egyptians (i.e., internal attribution) even when these phenomena stem from external factors. By clarifying these issues and providing accurate and objective explanations, the program sought to change this subjective tendency and to make the Israeli more cautious and less biased in his attributions and judgments. The intervention program included printed material presented in booklet form to the Israeli tourists at the start of their trip to Egypt.

Research Description

A quasi-experiment (Cook & Campbell, 1979) was designed in order to test the effects of combining the informational and contact approaches. The subjects were 483 Jewish Israeli tourists visiting Egypt on 31 organized tours. The tours were randomly divided into an experimental group (23 tours, $n = 352$) which was exposed to the intervention program and a control group (8 tours, $n = 131$) which was not exposed to it. There were no significant differences between the two groups in relation to their members' characteristics like sex, age, socioeconomic status, etc.

A questionnaire was constructed to assess the changes produced by the tour in the perception of Israelis regarding Egypt and Egyptians. The questionnaire comprised two kinds of scales: (a) a semantic-differential type scale which included a list of opposing characteristics such as friendly–unfriendly, peaceful–hostile, clean–dirty. The respondents were asked to evaluate "Egypt," "Egyptians," as well as "Egyptians as compared with Israelis" on the basis of the above characteristics; (b) questions regarding future prospects of Egyptian-Israeli relations, such as chances for permanent peace, willingness to compromise.

A factor analysis for the semantic differential scales revealed two factors: (a) social characteristics, such as polite, friendly, honest, pleasant, and peaceful; (b) characteristics indicating intelligence and competence, such as intellectual, efficient, and interesting. Factor scores were computed indicating, for each factor, the average of the subject's responses to all the questions. These scores ranged from 1 (positive) to 5 (negative).

A factor analysis for the questions on the prospect of peace yielded one factor. The scores for this ranged from 1 (positive) to 4 (negative). Thus, each subject received three scores, one for each of the three factors listed above, which will be labeled social, intellectual, and political.

Two identical versions of this questionnaire were developed, one for before and one for after the tour experience. They were identical except that the post-tour questionnaire added a few questions about satisfaction with the tour. The procedure included administering the "before" questionnaire to the experimental and control groups, carrying out the intervention program for the experimental group, and administering the "after" questionnaire. The "before" measures were administered during the bus ride from Israel to the Egyptian border, the "after" questionnaire upon the completion of the tour.

Results and Discussion

Effects of Contact Only

In order to assess attitude changes produced by the tour itself, i.e., contact per se, the difference between the "before" and "after" measures of the control group was examined. The data were analyzed for each of the three attitude factors.

Table 1. Mean attitude scores of experimental and control groups before and after the tour

Dimension	Control group (8 tours, $n = 131$)					Experimental group (23 tours, $n = 352$)				
	Before	After	Difference[c]	t	p	Before	After	Difference[c]	t	p
Intellectual[a]	3.06	3.33	−0.27	−7.50	0.001	3.09	3.20	−0.11	−5.28	0.001
Social[a]	2.10	1.83	0.27	6.52	0.001	2.18	1.85	0.33	13.61	0.001
Political[b]	2.11	2.04	0.07	1.15	n.s.	2.17	2.01	0.16	5.44	0.001

[a] Scores ranged from 1 (positive) to 5 (negative).
[b] Scores ranged from 1 (positive) to 4 (negative).
[c] Positive scores indicate a positive change following the tour, negative scores a negative change.

As can be seen in the "before–after" comparisons of the control group columns in Table 1, subjects changed negatively on the intellectual dimension and positively on the social dimension. No significant differences were found for the political dimension. The common denominator underlying these findings is that the change was in the same direction as the respondent's original attitude: when the group's original attitude was positive the direction of change was positive; and when the original attitude was negative the direction of change was negative. These results are consistent with the findings of Amir and Garti (1977), Brickman, Redfield, Harrison, and Crandall (1972), and Taylor and Koivumaki (1976). The findings can be interpreted in terms of motivational and cognitive processes underlying perception. Thus, one possible explanation for the above enhancement based on the cognitive factors of perception is that the obtained change is a result of selective perception which constitutes a reinforcement of the original attitude. The visit to Egypt is a mosaic of positive and negative experiences which may serve to strengthen earlier expectations. The Israeli tourist perceives the Egyptian reality through the lens of his original attitudes and is consequently biased in the same direction.

An alternative explanation for the results, based on motivational factors, may be derived from findings of Bizman and Amir (1982), who showed that the Israelis agree that they excel intellectually rather than socially, while the opposite holds true for the Arabs. Thus, the differential pattern of change in the two dimensions could reflect an accentuation of the Israelis' feeling of superiority in the intellectual dimension and of their relative "weakness" in the social domain.

Finally, of course, there remains the possibility that the Israeli is not a reality-distorter, but a realist and that the direction of change in his attitudes indeed reflects the reality he encounters. As described earlier, the Israeli visitor to Egypt is exposed throughout his trip primarily to negative aspects of the intellectual-competence realm of Egypt. This is likely to lead to attributions of backwardness and incompetence. On the other hand, as a tourist the Israeli is in frequent contact with service personnel who are polite, accommodating, and pleasant. Thus, he is positively impressed by the personal and social characteristics of the population he meets.

Still, it is difficult to determine which of the above alternatives accounts for the changes in the Israelis' attitudes towards the Egyptians.

Effect of Combining Contact and Information

To assess the effects of the experimental intervention, the difference between the "before" and "after" measures of the experimental group was examined. The data for this are presented in Table 1, in the experimental group column. Findings indicate a negative change on the intellectual dimension and a positive change on the social and political dimensions.

To assess the net effect of the intervention program we compared the differences in change between the control and the experimental groups. To this end a multivariate analysis of variance was performed consisting of two types of group (between) and three dimensions of attitude (within) with the appropriate before-measure of each dimension as a covariate. Table 1 presents the mean attitude scores of the two groups, before and after the tour, for the three dimensions, and the two columns on the right side of the table provide the results for the above analyses.

The analyses indicate that change had occurred as a result of the intervention. The main effect of group (intervention vs. no intervention) was significant, $F(1, 475) = 3.95$, $p < 0.05$, and the direction of change was congruent with the intervention: the experimental group exhibited more positive change than the control group. The interaction between attitude dimensions and group was significant, $F(2, 951) = 3.17$, $p < 0.05$, indicating differential changes on the three dimensions in the two groups. In order to specify these differences a one-way analysis of covariance was computed for each dimension. This analysis yielded a highly significant effect for the intellectual dimension, $F(1, 482) = 2.16$, $p < 0.0001$, indicating a more negative change in the control group (-0.27) as compared with the experimental group (-0.11). No significant differences were found for the other two dimensions.

This one-dimensional change is probably related to the fact that positive phenomena of the social dimension were experienced directly by both the experimental and control groups during the trip itself (i.e., the Egyptians are sociable, friendly, helpful), and the information provided regarding this dimension by the intervention did not exert additional effects. In contrast, on the intellectual dimension, the intervention provided the tourist with information that was different and more positive than that experienced on the trip. Thus, the control group subjects who were exposed to negative experiences in this direction evidenced a negative change, whereas the experimental group subjects who received additional positive inputs evidenced less of a negative change. The political issue was hardly evident during the tours and was not brought up in the manipulation and, indeed, no differences between the groups were found in this dimension.

In sum, then, even though the intervention was not effective enough to induce positive changes, it at least succeeded in moderating negative ones. Similar findings were recently obtained in another study on attitude change in ethnic relations (Ben-Ari, 1982).

It should be added that the above reported findings were consistent over time. A second "after" measure was administered to all subjects about 4 months after the initial measurement. No differences were found for the two "after" measures for all groups and dimensions, indicating that the results obtained immediately after the tours did not change over time.

Three additional questions were tested in relation to the above findings, namely, whether the results were connected to the individual's satisfaction from the tour, to his initial political attitude, or to any of a number of background variables.

With regard to the individual's satisfaction from the tour, we tested to what extent the changes obtained in the intervention group were related to the general satisfaction of the visitors with their trip, which could reflect some kind of a "halo effect." No correlation between the degree of satisfaction from the trip and each of the three attitude dimensions was found. Moreover, the experimental and control groups did not differ in the degree of their satisfaction with the trip.

In relation to the initial political attitudes we tested whether persons who scored positively on the political dimension, that is, who were relatively optimistic about the chances of resolving the Egyptian-Israeli conflict, changed more positively toward Egypt and Egyptians than subjects with negative scores on this dimension. The results showed no significant differences between these two kinds of subjects, indicating that the initial political attitude cannot be considered a factor in the process of attitude change.

In order to assess possible effects of various background variables, two-way analyses of variance with repeated measures were conducted. No significant effects were obtained for any of the variables tested.

Summary

The present study tested the "contact hypothesis" in the area of international tourism. As in other studies on ethnic contact, it was found that strong belief in interethnic contact must be qualified: intergroup contact per se does not guarantee positive attitude change. The study demonstrated that in order to increase the chances for positive results, the participants in the contact situation should be cognitively prepared for it. The preparation in this study took the form of an informational program supplied to the tourists prior to their contact experience. The results of the study show that combining information with contact can improve the contact results.

Examining the "contact approach" and the "information approach" to inducing change in ethnic attitudes of one ethnic group toward the other constitutes a novel approach in the area of tourism. Social science literature and research on tourism are primarily concerned with economic issues, with only some contributions from geographers, anthropologists, sociologists, and hardly any psychologists. Still, as tourism is a huge multinational enterprise involving people, one would expect more academic research, particularly in the behavioral sciences.

Research concerned with the social contact between tourists and their hosts has been predominantly interested in the tourists' impact on the host community (Pearce, 1982). In this area the interest is on the negative effects of tourism, such as disturbances in the social order and the stimulation of various social problems (e.g., begging, prostitution, crime), and on its positive effects, like creating new jobs, community modernization, and strengthening of cultural traditions. Even when the research deals with social perceptions and attitudes, the interest concentrates only on those of the hosts toward the tourists. From the tourists' point of view, touring is perceived as a means of leisure and enjoyment, but not as a vehicle for changing attitudes and perceptions.

In the present research the researchers tried to look at the contact between tourist and host as a social-psychological process, and to ask about the impact of such contact on the tourist's attitudes and perceptions regarding the host culture. In order to understand the general processes and forces which account for such an impact, interpersonal forces (like the context of the contact and the group membership of the participants) and intraindividual aspects (like attitudes, motives, and social character of the participants) operating in the encounter have to be taken into consideration. The question whether tourism will bring about understanding, empathy, and positive change in the tourists' perceptions and attitudes toward the host culture or will reinforce prevailing prejudices and stereotypes depends upon the characteristics of the forces that operate in the contact situation.

In the setting of the present study the interpersonal aspects mentioned above were not under the control of the researchers. On the other hand, some possibilities were available to intervene at the intraindividual level. To reach an optimal level for producing changes in ethnic attitudes and perceptions through intergroup contact, special information was provided to the Israeli tourist. This information emphasized positive (in the eyes of the Israelis) aspects of the Egyptian culture and matters common to Israelis and Egyptians, and prepared the tourists for different social situations which might prove to be unpleasant or tension-loaded. This was intended to reduce the salience of the cultural gap almost inevitable in such contact situations (Taft, 1977), to increase the enjoyment during the trips and the intergroup contact, as well as to facilitate the "positive presentation" of the Egyptian in the eyes of the Israeli.

The social setting of tourism may be particularly conducive to cognitive preparation by the provision of information, since the tourist enters the contact situation of his own volition and has a strong motivation to be exposed to new information and experiences. The setting of tourism can, therefore, be considered as an "unfreezing stage" according to Lewin's (1958) theory on change in attitude and perception. When unfreezing occurs, there is a possibility of adopting new plausible alternative beliefs inconsistent with the stored knowledge (Kruglanski & Ajzen, 1983), as this process "is determined by the ability to entertain new ideas and collect new information, the availability and salience of new information and the development of the motivation for validity" (Bar-Tal & Geva, 1986).

Considering tourism as a tool for social change still leaves us with many questions regarding the possible impact of various elements of the tour itself. For example, what are the effects of the tour guides, and how are they best prepared in order to serve as positive informational sources? Does it make a difference whether the tourist travels alone or within a group? To what extent is the group that one travels with relevant to the development of ingroup-outgroup perceptions and social comparison processes, thereby hinderling or facilitating positive changes in perceptions and attitudes? What are the specific effects of the type of information presented to the tourist throughout the tour? For instance, tourism often tends to emphasize the country's heritage by exhibiting outdated folklore and tradition, and not the positive aspects of the society, such as aspects of progress and humanity. In such a case, what image of the host country will be produced in the tourist's mind? Are the organizers of tours aware of the attitudes and perception that may be established after the tours?

Thus, it seems that there are still many open questions, and much research is needed regarding the different variables operating in the tourist setting which may be relevant to the issues raised here. The present study may serve as a starting point in this direction.

Today, when geographical distances among national and cultural groups are dramatically reduced and the number of visitors to foreign countries has drastically increased, international tourism provides an opportunity for closing the psychological gaps among them. The present study suggests that techniques can be developed to improve relations between two peoples that have until recently been enemies in a state of war. Even greater success may be expected when implementing such methods on peoples whose initial ethnic attitudes and interactions are not as negative as may have been the case in this study.

References

Allport, G. W. (1954). *The nature of prejudice*. Cambridge, MA: Addison-Wesley.

Amir, Y. (1969). Contact hypothesis in ethnic relations. *Psychological Bulletin, 71,* 319–342.

Amir, Y. (1976). The role of intergroup contact in change of prejudice and ethnic relations. In P. A. Katz (Ed.), *Towards the elimination of racism* (pp. 245–308). New York: Pergamon.

Amir, Y., & Ben-Ari, R. (1985). International tourism, ethnic contact and attitude change. *Journal of Social Issues, 41* (3), 105–115.

Amir, Y., Ben-Ari, R., Bizman, A., & Rivner, M. (1980). Contact between Israelis and Arabs: A theoretical evaluation of effects. *Journal of Cross-Cultural Psychology, 11,* 426–443.

Amir, Y., Ben-Ari, R., Bizman, A., & Rivner, M. (1982). Objective versus subjective aspects of interpersonal relations between Jews and Arabs. *Journal of Conflict Resolution, 26,* 485–506.

Amir, Y., & Garti, C. (1977). Situational and personal influences on attitude change following ethnic contact. *International Journal of Intercultural Relations, 1,* 58–75.

Ashmore, R. D. (1970). Solving the problem of prejudice. In B. E. Collins (Ed.), *Social psychology*. Reading, MA: Addison-Wesley.

Bar-Tal, D., & Geva, N. (1986). A cognitive basis of international conflicts. In S. Worchel & W. G. Austin (Eds.), *Psychology of intergroup relations*. Chicago: Nelson Hall.

Ben-Ari, R. (1982). *Satisfaction of interpersonal needs in ethnically mixed schools and change in intergroup relations*. Doctoral dissertation, Bar-Ilan University, Ramat-Gan, Israel.

Berelson, B., & Steiner, G. A. (1964). *Human behavior: An inventory of scientific findings*. New York: Harcourt, Brace & World.

Bizman, A., & Amir, Y. (1982). Mutual perception of Arabs and Jews in Israel. *Journal of Cross-Cultural Psychology, 13,* 461–469.

Bloom, L. (1971). *The social psychology of race relations*. London: Allen & Unwin.

Bolton, E. B. (1935). Effects of knowledge upon attitudes towards the Negro. *Journal of Social Psychology, 6,* 68–90.

Brewer, M. B., & Campbell, D. T. (1976). *Ethnocentrism and intergroup attitudes: East African evidence*. New York: Halsted.

Brickman, P., Redfield, J., Harrison, A. A., & Crandall, R. (1972). Drive and predisposition in the attitude effects of mere exposure. *Journal of Experimental Social Psychology, 8,* 31–44.

Brislin, R. W., Cushner, K., Cherrie, C., & Yong, M. (1986). *Intercultural interactions: A practical guide*. New York: Sage.

Byrne, D. (1969). Attitude and attraction. In L. Berkowitz (Ed.), *Advances in experimental and social psychology* (Vol. 4). New York: Academic.

Campbell, D. T. (1965). Ethnocentric and other altruistic motives. In D. Levine (Ed.), *Nebraska symposium on motivation* (Vol. 13, pp. 283–311). Lincoln: University of Nebraska Press.

Cook, S. W. (1962). The systematic analysis of socially significant events: A strategy for social research. *Journal of Social Issues, 18,* 66–84.

Cook, S. W. (1970). Motives in conceptual analysis of attitude-related behavior. In W. J. Arnold & D. Levine (Eds.), *Nebraska symposium on motivation, 1969*. Lincoln: University of Nebraska Press.

Cook, T., & Campbell, D. (1979). *Quasi-experimentation: Design and analysis issues for field setting*. Boston: Houghton Mifflin.

Cooper, E., & Dinerman, H. (1951). Analysis of the film, "Don't be a sucker": A study in communication. *Public Opinion Quarterly, 15,* 243–264.

Crawford, T. J. (1974). Sermons on racial tolerance and the parish neighborhood context. *Journal of Applied Social Psychology, 4,* 1–23.

Davis, E. E., & Fine, M. (1975). The effects of the findings of the US National Advisory Commission on Civil Disorders: An experimental study of attitude change. *Human Relations, 28,* 209-227.

Hamilton, D.L. (1979). A cognitive attributional analysis of stereotyping. In L.Berkowitz (Ed.), *Advances in experimental social psychology* (Vol.12). New York: Academic.

Harding, J., Proshansky, H., Kutner, B., & Chein, I. (1969). Prejudice and ethnic relations. In G.Lindzey & E.Aronson (Eds.), *The handbook of social psychology.* Reading, MA: Addison-Wesley.

Hofman, J.E. (1977). Identity and intergroup perceptions in Israel. *International Journal of Intercultural Relations, 1,* 79-102.

Hovland, C.I., Harvey, O., & Sherif, M. (1957). Assimilation and contrast effect in communication and attitude change. *Journal of Abnormal and Social Psychology, 55,* 242-252.

Kelley, H.H. (1972). Causal schemata in the attribution process. In E.E.Jones et al. (Eds.), *Attribution: Perceiving the causes of behavior.* New Jersey: General Learning.

Kruglanski, A.W., & Ajzen, I. (1983). Bias and error in human judgment. *European Journal of Social Psychology, 13,* 1-44.

Landis, D., Hope, R.C., & Day, H.R. (1984). Training for desegregation in the military. In N.Miller & M.B.Brewer (Eds.), *Groups in contact: The psychology of desegregation.* Orlando, FL: Academic.

Lewin, K. (1958). Group decision and social change. In E.Maccoby, T.M.Newcomb, & E.L.Hartley (Eds.), *Readings in social psychology* (pp.197-211). New York: Holt, Rinehart & Winston.

Miller, N. (1981). Changing views about the effects of school desegregation. *Brown* then and now. In M.B.Brewer & B.E.Collins (Eds.), *Scientific inquiry and the social sciences.* San Francisco: Jossey-Bass.

Murphy, G., & Likert, R. (1938). *Public opinions and the individual.* New York: Russell & Russell.

Myrdal, G. (1944). *An American dilemma.* New York: Harper & Row.

Nettler, G. (1946). The relationship between attitude and information concerning the Japanese in America. *American Sociological Review, 11,* 177-191.

Newcomb, T.M. (1961). *The acquaintance process.* New York: Holt, Rinehart & Winston.

Pearce, P.L. (1982). *The social psychology of tourist behaviour.* Oxford: Pergamon.

Rabbie, J.M., & Horwitz, M. (1969). Arousal of ingroup-outgroup bias by a chance win or loss. *Journal of Personality and Social Psychology, 13,* 269-277.

Rokeach, M. (Ed.) (1960). *The open and closed mind.* New York: Basic Books.

Secord, P.F., & Backman, C.W. (1974). *Social psychology.* New York: McGraw-Hill.

Sherif, M., Harvey, O.J., White, B.J., Hood, W.R., & Sherif, C. (1961). *Intergroup conflict and cooperation: The robber's cave experiment.* Norman, OK: University Book Exchange.

Sherif, M., & Sherif, C.W. (1969). *Social psychology.* New York: Harper.

Sinha, A.K.P., & Upadhyaya, O.P. (1960). Change and persistence in the stereotype of university students towards different ethnic groups during Sino-Indian border dispute. *Journal of Social Psychology, 52,* 31-39.

Stephan, W.G., & Stephan, C.W. (1984). The role of ignorance in intergroup relations. In N.Miller & M.B.Brewer (Eds.), *Groups in contact: The psychology of desegregation.* Orlando, FL: Academic.

St.John, N.S. (1975). *School desegregation: Outcomes for children.* New York: Wiley.

Taft, R. (1977). Coping with unfamiliar cultures. In N.Warren (Ed.), *Studies in cross-cultural psychology* (Vol.1). London: Academic.

Tajfel, H. (1981). *Human groups and social categories: Studies in social psychology.* Cambridge: Cambridge University Press.

Tajfel, H., & Dawson, J.L. (Eds.) (1965). *Disappointed guests.* London: Oxford University Press.

Taylor, S.E., Fiske, S.T., Etcoff, N.L., & Ruderman, A.J. (1978). Categorical and contextual bases of person memory and stereotyping. *Journal of Personality and Social Psychology, 36,* 778-793.

Taylor, S.E., & Koivumaki, J.H. (1976). The perception of self and others: Acquaintanceship, affect, and actor-observer differences. *Journal of Personality and Social Psychology, 33,* 403-408.

Triandis, H.C. (1975). Cultural training, cognitive complexity and interpersonal attitudes. In R. Brislin, S. Bochner, & W. Lonner (Eds.), *Cross-cultural perspectives on learning*. New York: Wiley.

Wagner, U., & Schoenbach, P. (1984). Links between educational status and prejudice: Ethnic attitudes in West Germany. In N. Miller & M.B. Brewer (Eds.), *Groups in contact: The psychology of desegregation*. Orlando, FL: Academic.

Williams, R.M., Jr. (1947). *The reduction of intergroup tensions: A survey of research on problems of ethnic, racial, and religious group relations*. New York: Social Science Research Council.

Chapter 10

Familiarity May Breed Contempt: The Impact of Student Exchange on National Stereotypes and Attitudes

Wolfgang Stroebe, Andrea Lenkert, and Klaus Jonas

Introduction

To justify the inclusion of a chapter on the impact of student exchange on national stereotypes and attitudes in a book on conflict, two assumptions have to be made that are deceptively plausible. First, it has to be accepted that stereotypes and attitudes play a causal role in creating, maintaining, or aggravating intergroup conflicts. Second, it has to be assumed that student exchange typically changes stereotypes in ways that improve the sojourners' attitudes towards the host nation and thus serves a function in conflict reduction.

The first assumption is widely shared by social scientists (e.g., Deutsch, 1973; Klineberg, 1954; Sherif, 1967). Although it is emphasized that stereotypes are products, not initial causes, of intergroup conflict and hostility, it is generally assumed that negative stereotypes and attitudes tend to bias future interactions between members of different groups who possess these stereotypes. According to Cantril (1950, cited by Sherif, 1967, p. 26), a panel of social scientists and psychiatrists assembled by UNESCO some decades ago even went so far as to consider stereotypes and prejudice as a contributor to modern war. They agreed that "myth, traditions and symbols for national pride handed down from one generation to another" are among the factors conducive to "modern wars between nations and groups of nations" (Cantril, 1950, p. 18). More moderately, Sherif (1967) argued that "group prejudice and derogatory images of other peoples, though products of historical processes forming part of people's cultural heritage, may exert a fateful influence on the ongoing process between groups" (1967, p. 26).

The stepwise progression from intergroup conflict to negative stereotypes and attitudes, which then maintain continued intergroup hostility, was repeatedly demonstrated in the classic set of studies conducted by Sherif and his co-workers (Sherif, Harvey, White, Hood, & Sherif, 1961). In these field experiments, newly formed groups of boys developed negative outgroup stereotypes after a conflict had been initiated between the groups. Once intergroup hostility had been aroused, even meeting in the most pleasant contact situations (e.g., going to the movies, eating in the same dining room) were merely used as occasions for the rival groups to berate and attack each other. Although such open signs of intergroup hostility may often be suppressed by situational constraints, intergroup stereotypes are likely to affect future interactions by attributional biases (see Hewstone, this volume).

The results of Sherif's studies suggest, however, that it may be somewhat naive to expect that interpersonal or intergroup contact will automatically lead to an improvement in intergroup attitudes and stereotypes. This has been recognized by most researchers in the area (e.g., Allport, 1954; Amir, 1969; Cook & Selltiz, 1955). Thus, Cook (1969, 1984; Cook & Selltiz, 1955), who conducted a number of impressive laboratory and field studies in interracial settings to investigate the effect of social contact on racial stereotypes and attitudes, described five conditions under which intergroup contact is likely to improve attitudes. Favorable attitude change can be facilitated by intergroup contact when (a) participants from both groups have equal status; (b) the member of the outgroup has characteristics which disconfirm previously held negative stereotypes (e.g., a fun-loving, easy-going German); (c) the contact situation has "high acquaintance potential" (i.e., the situation provides an opportunity for people to "get to know" one another as individual persons); (d) contact takes place in a situation in which social norms encourage friendly association; and finally, but perhaps most importantly, (e) the situation encourages cooperation between members of different groups. Cook (1984) summarized a great deal of empirical evidence to demonstrate that, given these favorable conditions, interracial contact tended to improve interracial attitudes and stereotypes. Similar points were raised by Amir (1969; see also Ben-Ari & Amir, this volume) in his influential review of research on the contact hypothesis (for a critical assessment of the contact hypothesis from an intergroup perspective, see Hewstone & Brown, 1986).

This set of favorable conditions should be comforting to any proponent of student exchange, since the exchange situation seems to have many of the characteristics likely to facilitate favorable attitude change. Thus, universities in most countries offer a setting that is egalitarian, has a high acquaintance potential, and social norms that encourage friendly association. While the study situation is not necessarily characterized by a cooperative reward structure, neither does it seem to be competitive.

In assessing the exchange situation in terms of the characteristics outlined by Cook (e.g. 1984), it should also be remembered that interracial contact was used to change the attitudes of individuals who had often been specifically chosen for their *prejudiced* attitudes. In contrast, students who choose to spend a year in a particular country are unlikely to have negative attitudes towards that country. Thus, the contact situation of exchange students is typically more favorable than that encountered by the participants in the studies conducted by Cook (1984).

A Review of the Literature: Some Disappointing Findings

In view of the excellent reasons why student exchange should facilitate an improvement in attitudes towards a host country, it is sobering to realize that this is not the typical finding of the numerous investigations into exchange students' attitudes (for reviews see Klineberg, 1966; de Sola Pool, 1965; Spaulding & Flack, 1976). Thus, Selltiz and Cook (1962; Selltiz, Christ, Havel, & Cook, 1963) reject the assumption that getting to know people of another country will increase attraction towards them as "oversimplified and overly optimistic." This assumption is basic, however, to the expectation that "exchange-of-persons programs" will increase international good will.

In two longitudinal studies conducted on samples of several hundred foreign students in the United States of America in 1954 and 1955, Selltiz et al. (1963) reported a slight but significant deterioration in the foreign students' attitudes towards the United States. "The summary evaluation index, made up of students' responses to all the evaluation questions, showed a slight downward shift – that is, a decrease in favorableness during the year – in both studies" (p. 188). Similar conclusions were drawn earlier by Loomis and Schuler (1948) who used a longitudinal design to study the impact of a year's training in agriculture in the United States on students from Latin American countries. These authors concluded that "apprentice trainees from the Latin American countries after one year's stay have, in certain significant areas, less favorable attitudes towards the USA and its culture than they had on arrival" (Loomis & Schuler, 1948, p. 33).

That this kind of deterioration in evaluations of the host population among exchange students is not restricted to foreign students in the United States has been demonstrated by Klineberg and Hull (1979) in the most extensive study in this area to date. With an international group of collaborators, they conducted a questionnaire survey of 2,536 students from a wide variety of countries who were enrolled in institutions of postsecondary education in Brazil, Canada, the Federal Republic of Germany, Hong Kong, India, Iran, Japan, Kenya, the United Kingdom, and the United States. Although they collected some longitudinal data on a small subsample of their students, they do not present any attitude data from this longitudinal analysis. Thus, information on attitude "change" had to be based on a comparison of the foreign students' attitudes towards the local people at the time of the survey, and their *recollections* of what their attitudes had been before their arrival. On the basis of these data, Klineberg and Hull (1979) reported that attitudes "were on the whole friendly on arrival, but [became] slightly *less* so on the average after a period of residence in nine out of our eleven countries" (p. 190). In the other two countries (Japan, Kenya), attitudes did not markedly improve but stayed approximately the same. While the fact that the overwhelming majority of these students remembered their initial attitude as being more favorable than their present one can certainly be interpreted as an indication of disenchantment with their hosts, it does not necessarily mean that initial attitudes were really more positive.

The same problem arises in interpreting findings from a much smaller study conducted by Hafeez Zaidi (1975) of 121 foreign students, mainly from African and Asian countries, who studied in Karachi (Pakistan). This is one of the few studies of Asian and African students sojourning in an Asian country. Hafeez Zaidi (1975) gives the following summary of his findings on the impact of the sojourn on attitudes toward the host population: "Their image of the people of Pakistan as a religious, honest, and brave people may also undergo some change in the process of adjustment to the realities of the situation. Some of their responses indicate that Pakistanis are perceived as changing for the better, but on the whole their assessment is unfavorable. They find Pakistanis to be shrewd, selfish, unsocial, uncooperative, violent, and not true Muslims" (p. 126). Although this conclusion reads as if it were derived from longitudinal data (and indeed it derives from comparisons of the images foreign students hold of Pakistanis before arrival in Pakistan and after), the description of the procedure suggests that interviews were conducted at only one point in time and that the information about images that existed before arrival was collected retrospectively.

There is some evidence suggesting that studying in foreign countries results in a more positive attitude, but interpretations of such findings are also not unproblematic. For example, Riegel (1953), in a widely cited paper, reported a comparison of attitudes of 150 former Belgian exchangees to the United States with a group of "135 similar Belgians with similar professions and social status who had never sojourned in the United States" (p. 320). Although he concluded that "personal popularity of Americans was greater among former exchangees than among other Belgians" (p. 322), it is difficult to assess the validity of this inference in the absence of data or statistical tests. Riegel's own statement that "it was felt that an active or latent hope of being selected again, or of receiving other forms of American favor or patronage, affected the testimony of many grantees" (p. 321) does not greatly increase one's trust in the validity of his findings. Finally, it could be argued that his comparison group was inadequate. It seems plausible that individuals who choose to apply for a grant to visit the United States hold more favorable attitudes towards the States even before their visit than a matched group of individuals who did not make this choice.

Since Riegel (1953) interviewed his sample after their return to their home country, the discrepancy between his findings and those of the studies reported earlier could be construed as an indication of changes over time in attitudes towards the former hosts. It would be plausible that after students return home, their views and feeling about the host country become more positive. Since judgments about the host country are likely to be based on a comparison with the students' own country, their return to the reality of their home country could lead to a change in their evaluation of the exchange experience. However, if this assumption were to account for the results of the Riegel (1953) study, one would expect a positive association between attitude and the time period since return. Contrary to this, Riegel found that students were most favorable towards the host country immediately after their return.

Another widely held assumption about time changes in attitudes towards the host nation has become known as the "U curve of adjustment." According to this hypothesis, foreign students go through a cycle in their feelings towards the host country. The beginning of their sojourn is characterized by a "honeymoon phase" which lasts for approximately 6 months (Lysgaard, 1955). This phase of enthusiasm is followed by a period of disenchantment and depression. Once this "crisis of adjustment," assumed to last for more than a year, has been overcome, the visitor begins to feel better adjusted and more integrated. As a consequence of this improvement, the period of relatively negative feelings is followed by a return to a more favorable attitude (see, e.g., Chang, 1973; Lysgaard, 1955; Selltiz & Cook, 1962, Sewell & Davidsen, 1961). Although there is some discrepancy in the timing of this "low" (e.g., Coelho, 1958; Lysgaard, 1955; Morris 1960), the end of a 1-year period comes near the bottom of the "U" according to most estimates. Since exchange visits are frequently limited to one year, this hypothesis could account for the deterioration in attitudes observed in a great number of studies (e.g., Loomis & Schuler, 1948; Hafeez Zaidi, 1975; Selltiz & Cook, 1962).

Although some of the early studies (e.g., Deutsch & Won, 1963; Lysgaard, 1955; Sewell & Davidsen, 1961) claimed support for the hypothesis, more recent evaluations of the evidence have considered it weak (Breitenbach, 1970) and inconclusive (Spaulding & Flack, 1976). Furthermore, Klineberg and Hull (1979), who broke down their sample by length of sojourn in several ways and looked at variables such as "number of problems reported" and "personal depression" as well as attitudes towards the host population, found no support for the U-curve hypothesis.

In conclusion, the majority of studies on the impact of foreign exchange on stereotypes of, and liking for, the host nation seem to challenge the expectation that meeting and "getting to know" people of another country will increase attraction towards them. This conclusion has to be qualified by the reservation that in an area in which the "one shot case study" (Campbell & Stanley, 1966) done retrospectively is still widely used as evidence, even the better studies are not unproblematic. For example, even though exchange students are a group that is (self-) selected for its positive attitudes towards the host country and thus liable to regression effects in repeated measures designs (Campbell & Stanley, 1966), the longitudinal studies described earlier did not control for regression. In view of these methodological weaknesses, it was decided to conduct a study with the objective of examining the impact of foreign exchange on attitudes toward the host nation under more stringent methodological conditions.

American Students in France and Germany: An Empirical Study

Sample and Design

The participants in our study were 70 American exchange students of the California State University who in 1983 studied either in France (University of Aix-en-Provence) or Germany (Universities of Tübingen and Heidelberg). This constituted 46% of the relevant cohorts of exchange students from California State University. To assess the impact of their sojourn on attitudes and stereotypes, approximately half of our subjects – those on a short stay in Germany (Gs: $n = 18$) and France (Fs: $n = 16$) – were interviewed within a few weeks of their arrival, while the other half, on long stays (Gl: $n = 14$; Fl: $n = 22$), were approached near the end of their 1-year stay. Since most of the questionnaires used in this study had been developed in a large-scale survey of more than 1400 American students, which assessed their stereotypes and attitudes towards Europe and Europeans (Stapf, Stroebe, & Jonas, 1986), a comparison with these American data was possible in order to evaluate the extent to which the exchange students different from the typical American student.

Our study has a number of features which distinguish it from most previous research. First by taking measurements from comparable groups at the beginning and at the end of their sojourn, the impact of student exchange on views about the host nation can be assessed, even though this is not a longitudinal study. Second, by having participants from one university study in two different countries, one can hope to separate aspects that are general to the exchange situation from those which are specific to staying in a particular country. Furthermore, each group can serve as control group for the other. Finally, by measuring attitudes and stereotypes towards 14 nations (West Germans, French, Americans, Swedish, English, Polish, Japanese, Italians, East Germans, Spanish, Dutch, Russians, Canadians, Swiss) it is possible to clarify whether the sojourn affects only attitudes and stereotypes towards the host nation or has a more general impact on attitudes towards other countries, including the students' own. (These nations were used as stimuli because they had also been included in the Stapf et al. [1986] study.)

Objectives

The study was conducted to clarify three questions:

1. Do national stereotypes (i.e., the traits people attribute to members of different nations) change as a result of the sojourn? We were interested not only in the impact of the exchange on stereotypes of the host nation, but also in the more general effect of the sojourn on stereotypes of other European nations and on the stereotype these American students have of their own nation.
2. Does the extended stay abroad lead to attitude change? Again, we were interested not only in attitudes towards the host nation but also in a more general change in attitudes towards other nations. In addition, attitudes were measured towards several relevant aspects of the exchange situation (e.g., culture, university system, food).
3. What are the variables or processes that mediate the expected change in attitudes? As the impact of exchange was studied from the perspective of the "contact hypothesis," the amount and quality of interactions with members of the host nation was a key factor to assess here.

Measures

Since the classic study by Katz and Braly (1933), it has been customary to assess stereotypes using lists of trait descriptions. Subjects are asked to select those traits which to them seem to be most typical of the group in question. Implementing Brigham's (1971) critique of the Katz and Braly method, the present study assessed stereotypes by asking participants to indicate the percentage of members of a given national group that are thought to have each of a number of listed traits. In addition, students were asked to write down the most positive and most negative traits of their host nation.

More global than the study of specific trait attributions is the assessment of the dimensions individuals use to judge the similarities and differences between different nations. These dimensions were investigated by having students rate the similarity of all possible pairs of stimulus nations and by analyzing these ratings by methods of multidimensional scaling (MDS; model: individual differences). Further MDS analyses were conducted on the similarity ratings of the four groups (Fs, Fl, Gs, Gl) for some indication of whether the sojourn affected these students' "cognitive map" of Europe.

Attitudes towards members of the host nation, as well as towards other nations, were measured by two different methods. First, the percentage of members of a given nation thought of as "likeable" was used as a measure of attraction. In addition, subjects had to rate a subset of nations (Germans, French, English) on a seven-point positive to negative rating scale. The English were included here as an additional control, to have the nation of a country which was not an exchange country for either group. Similar rating scales were used to assess subjects' attitudes towards various relevant aspects of these three countries (e.g., culture, country as a setting for a student exchange, university system).

Since the study focused on the impact of social contact with the host population, this aspect was assessed extensively. Students approached at the end of their sojourn were asked to decribe their lodging (e.g., private room, dormitory). In addition they had to rate the extent of contact with American students and students of the host nation during the sojourn, the difficulty of achieving contact with members of the host nation, whether they would have liked these contacts to be better, and, finally, the perceived attitudes of the host students towards them.

Thus, the questionnaire used in this study contained the following measures: (a) similarity judgments of the 14 stimulus nations, requiring subjects to rate the extent of similarity for each possible pair of nationalities; (b) assessment of students' stereotypes of 14 nations through a list of traits; (c) free-response descriptions of stereotypes; (d) measurement of attitudes towards the Germans and the French (and the English) as well as towards various features of these three countries; (e) questions about biographical information, living arrangements, amount and quality of contacts with nationals from the host country, and an assessment of the value of the exchange experience.

Procedure

These questionnaires were typically filled out under supervision of a research associate. The initial contact with potential participants was made by a letter sent to them 3 weeks before the data were to be collected. The letter described the study as one concerned with "the impact on individuals of studying abroad." To make it clear that the researchers were neither associated with the exchange program (though obviously working with the permission of the program director) nor members of the host nation, the stationery of a German university was used for the letters to students in France and of a French university to students in Germany. Data were then collected at the various university towns by a German investigator in France and a French investigator in Germany to keep conditions comparable.

Findings

Cognitive Structure

An analysis of the similarity ratings by MDS was conducted to indicate the dimensions of the "cognitive map" which these American students use to represent similarities and differences between the 14 stimulus nations. In addition, MDS analyses were carried out for the four subsamples separately to show whether these maps changed in the course of the sojourn. After all, it is not implausible that, after spending a year abroad, students use different dimensions to represent the various stimulus nations.

The MDS (ALSCAL; Young & Lewyckyj, 1981), based on similarity ratings of the total sample, resulted in three dimensions. If one attempts an intuitive interpretation of these dimensions, then dimension 1 (Fig. 1, horizontal axis) seems to reflect some kind of *political,* East-West dimension, with the Eastern European nations to the left, the Western nations to the right. Dimension 2 (Fig. 1, vertical axis), with the Spanish, Italians, and French separated from the other nations, suggests a temperament dimension, with the more emotional nations at one end and the less emotional at the other. (No plausible interpretation could be found for dimension 3, which is therefore not depicted here.)

The use of stereotype ratings offers a more objective method of interpreting the dimensions of the MDS (Wish, Deutsch, & Biener, 1970). Since the list of trait descriptions employed to measure stereotypes contains traits such as "emotional" and "passionate," one can use the ratings to check the intuitive interpretation of dimension 2 by correlating the rank-order of the nations on this dimension with their rank-order according to their ratings as "emotional" and "passionate." The finding that those two traits show the highest correlation (emotional: 0.80; passionate: 0.75) with the rank-order of the different nations on dimension 2 indicates that our interpretation has been quite valid. For dimension 1 the highest correlating traits are "open-minded" (0.86), "individualistic" (0.78), and "materialistic" (0.78). Since the trait list did not contain any

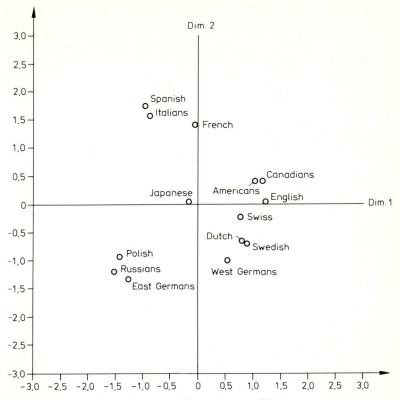

Fig. 1. Multidimensional scaling configuration (dimensions 1 and 2)

political terms, the East-West interpretation of this dimension could not be validated in this study. However, additional data collected by Stapf et al. (1986, p. 94) tend to support the interpretation of this dimension in terms of an East-West polarity.

The most interesting question, however, from the perspective of the present study, concerns the impact of the sojourn on these cognitive maps. Do these cognitive maps become more differentiated when students have lived for a year in Europe and/or do subjects use different dimensions? There is little evidence in our data that the length of sojourn or the choice of country had any impact on cognitive structure. When MDS analyses were computed separately for the four groups, each had 3 substantive dimensions, and when correlations of the orders of the nations on these three dimensions were compared across samples, the results were highly consistent. In view of the small size of these subsamples, this consistency was particularly surprising.

Stereotypes

Stereotypes were assessed by asking subjects to indicate the percentage of members of a given national group that were thought to possess each of a number of listed traits. Table 1 presents the ratings of the Germans and the French by the two groups of students who stayed in each of the two countries. For each group, the five adjectives with the highest ratings are set in bold face as the traits considered most typical for that nation.

In view of the small sample size, it is comforting that four of the five traits (efficient, industrious, intelligent, family-oriented) which the Gs group felt were most typical of the Germans were also seen as most characteristic of the Germans by the large sample of American students surveyed by Stapf et al. (1986). This suggests that the stereotype of the Germans held by the Gs group is widely shared by American students. Similarly, three of the top five traits used by the Fs group to describe the French (enjoy life, emotional, intelligent) were also in the top group in the Stapf et al. study.

Table 1. American exchange students' stereotypes towards their host nation by length of sojourn (percentage ratings)

	Germans		French	
	Short stay (Gs) %	Long stay (Gl) %	Short stay (Fs) %	Long stay (Fl) %
Intelligent	**77.7**	**72.2**	66.2	**67.2**
Cultivated	67.7	64.6	68.7	**67.2**
Outgoing	47.7	39.2	56.2	41.2
Religious	65.8	55.7	61.2	47.2
Conforming	**76.6**	**76.0**	54.8	57.5
Arrogant	50.0	50.0	58.7	**70.5**
Family-oriented	**76.6**	65.1	**74.6**	65.2
Honest	73.8	**81.1**	**69.5**	57.0
Enjoy life	62.1	56.9	**72.1**	57.1
Conservative	66.3	61.2	59.6	56.1
Egoistical	52.7	57.3	64.3	**74.9**
Individualistic	45.8	35.7	67.1	49.8
Ambitious	69.7	68.9	61.5	49.2
Materialistic	68.0	**73.0**	69.2	**70.5**
Friendly	56.5	47.6	60.2	40.7
Industrious	**78.3**	**75.0**	66.5	49.6
Emotional	45.2	43.9	**69.3**	50.3
Competitive	75.5	65.5	63.2	55.3
Traditional	71.3	65.3	**74.3**	60.9
Scientifically-minded	71.3	66.7	59.6	42.8
Passionate	46.9	35.7	69.2	48.6
Efficient	**79.1**	71.3	63.1	40.2
Hostile	36.6	27.7	29.4	51.8
Likable	65.6	56.0	67.6	42.5
Open-minded	46.1	42.8	61.8	40.9

The most interesting question in the context of this study concerns the impact of the sojourn on stereotypes of the host nation. To test whether the exchange visit resulted in an improvement or deterioration in the stereotypes held of the host nation, the trait list was divided into sets of positive, neutral, and negative adjectives. This subdivision was based on desirability ratings of these trait adjectives by a sample of American students. A comparison of the German stereotype of students who had just arrived in Germany (Gs) with those of the group (Gl) who had been there for nearly a year did not indicate any significant differences in the extent to which these two groups felt that positive, neutral, or negative traits were typical of the Germans. With regard to the French stereotype, however, there were significant differences between the Fl and the Fs groups for all three categories (all significant differences referred to in this chapter are significant at least at the 5% level of significance [two-tailed]). Compared to the students who had been in France for only a short time, students who had lived there for a year thought that the positive traits and the neutral traits were less typical of the French, while the negative traits were more typical. Thus, while an extended stay in Germany had little impact on the stereotypes students held of the Germans, a year in France led to a significant deterioration in the stereotypes held of the French.

The analysis of the free-response descriptions given by these students of the French and the Germans resulted in a comparable pattern. While the Gs group did not differ significantly from the Gl students in the frequency with which they assigned positive, neutral, or negative traits to the Germans, there was a significant difference in the French stereotype of the Fs and Fl subjects. Compared to the students who had just arrived in France, the students who had stayed there for nearly a year assigned half as many positive and twice as many negative traits to the French. The most frequently mentioned negative traits were "unfriendly," "rude," "arrogant," "cold," and "lazy." These reactions correspond closely to those reported by Klineberg and Hull (1979) for the international group of exchange students interviewed longitudinally in their study.

It has often been suggested (e.g., Church, 1982; Selltiz & Cook, 1962) that extended sojourns lead to more "international outlook" and a reduction in "ethnocentrism." Although it seems plausible that, in addition to changing beliefs about the host nation, spending a year in Europe should have some effect on students' beliefs about the traits that are characteristic of other European nations, a comparison of the long-term and the short-term groups with regard to their stereotypes of a sample of other European nations (e.g., Italians, East Germans, Swedes, Poles) resulted in only one significant change out of 36 tested.

There was also little support for the assumption that the sojourn led to a reduction in "ethnocentrism" or, more generally, to a change in the stereotype these students hold of their own nation. Thus, the same top four traits (friendly, outgoing, materialistic, competitive) of their own nation appeared in the list of top five traits of all four groups. The fifth trait was "industrious" in three lists, and "ambitious" in the fourth. There were also no significant differences between the short-term and long-term groups in their ratings of positive, neutral, and negative traits as being typical of their fellow Americans.

178   Wolfgang Stroebe et al.

There is one general effect, though, due to length of sojourn. The Gl and Fl groups seem to be more reluctant to make stereotype judgments than the Gs and Fs groups. Students who had spent a year in Europe rated the percentage of people of a given nation who possessed a particular trait consistently lower than students who had been assessed immediately after arrival. This change occurred for nations that were visited as well as for those that were not, and affected positive as well as negative traits. It is interesting that, while the percentage ratings were lowered, the stereotype profile seems to have stayed essentially the same. For example, the stereotype of the English of the Fs and Fl groups show a correlation of $r = 0.88$, even though the Fl group gave lower ratings on 20 out of 25 traits. The corresponding correlation for the Gs and Gl groups is $r = 0.82$, although the Gl group rated the percentage of English that possessed a given trait lower for 19 out of 25 adjectives.

In summary, while spending a year in France seems to have resulted in a significant change of the French stereotype towards a more negative image, a comparable sojourn in Germany had little effect on students' stereotype of the Germans. Furthermore, the year in Europe did not result in any major reassessment of the traits these students felt were characteristic of various European nations, nor did it have an impact on autostereotypes (i.e., the traits these students believed to be most characteristic of the Americans). It did, however, make students more careful in giving stereotype judgments.

Attitudes

Table 2 presents the attitudes of the short- and long-term groups towards their hosts, their host country, and some other attitude objects relevant to the exchange situation. It is apparent that the sojourn had a negative impact on attitudes towards both host countries. However, this change appeared to be more

Table 2. American exchange students' attitudes towards various aspects of their host country by length of soujourn

	Germans		French	
	Short stay (Gs)	Long stay (Gl)	Short stay (Fs)	Long stay (Fl)
People[a] (likeability)	65.60	56.00	67.60	42.50
People[b] (attitudes)	5.56	4.86	4.94	3.50
Country[b] (general)	5.89	5.43	5.87	4.18
Country[b] (for student exchange)	5.78	6.14	5.87	4.82
Culture[b]	5.61	5.57	5.69	4.76
Food[b]	4.39	4.43	5.62	5.82
University system[b]	4.88	3.64	3.69	2.43

[a] Percentage of likeable people in a given country (range: 0–100)
[b] Attitude ratings: higher numbers indicate more positive attitudes (range: 1–7)

marked for the attitudes towards the French rather than the Germans. Thus, the Fl group rated the French lowest in likeability of all nations, lower even than the Russians and East Germans, who typically come last in these popularity contests. But although, descriptively, the impact of the sojourn seems to have been more negative on attitudes towards the French than the Germans, two-factor analyses of variance (country × length of stay) resulted only in significant main effects, namely for country (the French being rated more negatively) and length of stay (the host nation being rated more negatively after a long rather than a short stay). There was no significant interaction. To check whether the impact of the sojourn on attitudes is limited to the host nations, t-tests were carried out on the differences in attitudes towards the French and the English of the Gs and Gl group and on the differences in attitudes towards the Germans and the English of the Fs and Fl groups. None of these differences even approached statistical significance.

The ANOVAs conducted on attitudes towards other aspects of the exchange situation suggest that students are quite discriminating in their evaluations. Thus, French food is considered better than German food and this attitude remains stable over time. On the other hand, the French University system is considered worse than the German, but attitudes towards both deteriorate over time. There is also a deterioration in attitudes towards France and Germany as countries (but not as countries for student exchange). This effect seems to be mainly due to a negative change in attitudes towards France ($p <$ 0.06 for the interaction of country × length of stay). As a country for student exchange, Germany was rated even slightly more positive at the end of the sojourn while France was rated more negative. This interaction reached statistical significance in a two-factor ANOVA (country × length of stay). It is interesting to note that changes in attitudes towards these aspects were again limited to the country which had been visited. Thus, length of sojourn had no significant impact on these attitudes with regard to England or on attitudes towards France of the group that stayed in Germany and towards Germany of the group that studied in France.

To summarize, then, the attitude findings show a fairly differentiated pattern. While attitudes towards the host nation and its people are on the whole more negative among students who stay in France rather than Germany, this is not true for all aspects of the exchange setting. Thus, there is no significant difference in attitudes towards German and French culture and French food is considered better than German food.

Mediating Variables

Most researchers in the area of student exchange agree that the number, variety, and depth of social encounters with members of the host nation is the most important variable related to the sojourners' adjustment (e. g., Church, 1982; Klineberg & Hull, 1979; Selltiz & Cook, 1962). For exchange students, the opportunity to establish contacts with members of the host nationality will depend to some extent on living arrangements during their stay abroad. Thus, students who live in dormitories should have greater opportunity to meet students from the host nation than individuals who rent their own apartment.

Our data suggest that living arrangements in Germany offered greater opportunities for contact than those in France. Thus, students in Germany had mostly rooms in dormitories, while those in France typically rented apartments, which they often shared with other Americans. It is thus hardly surprising that American students in France reported significantly greater difficulties than those in Germany in establishing contacts with both student and nonstudent members of the host nation.

To facilitate positive attitude change towards the host population, there should not only be contact, but contact that is experienced as pleasant by these American students. This is unlikely to happen, however, if the hosts are perceived as prejudiced and unsympathetic towards Americans. Again, it is the French students who are seen as holding significantly more unfriendly attitudes towards Americans than the German students, although there is room for improvement in the Germans' attitudes as well.

To summarize, then, the analysis of contact opportunities revealed differences between France and Germany which could go some way towards accounting for the pattern of stereotype and attitude findings. American students who stay in Germany are more likely than those in France to live in a dormitory. However, it may not only be the greater opportunity to establish contacts with students of the host nation which accounts for the greater favorability of the German stereotype, but also the fact that German students are attributed a somewhat more positive attitude towards Americans.

Summary and conclusions

The findings of this study are interesting for two reasons, namely, both the changes in attitudes and stereotypes that were observed and the changes that were not. To begin with the first: consistent with the findings of research reviewed earlier, there was no evidence of any improvement in these students' attitudes or stereotypes towards their host population. On the contrary, after spending a year in France or Germany, students liked their host nation (whether French or German) less than before, an effect which seems to have been somewhat more marked with regard to the French than the Germans. Students who had spent a year in France also held more negative stereotypes towards the French than students who had just arrived in the country.[1] This change in stereotypes was apparent in both students' answers to the trait list and their free responses. A year in Germany, on the other hand, did not lead to a significant deterioration in students' stereotypes of the Germans.

---

1 Since the "French" sample consisted only of American students who studied at the University of Aix-en-Provence, it could be argued that our findings reflect factors that are specific to Aix rather than France. However, the fact that students interviewed by Klineberg and Hull (1979) described the French in very similar terms to those used by the students comprising this sample suggests that our findings are more general.

Although these changes are interesting to a social psychologist, we would argue that the changes that one would have expected to occur (but apparently did not) are even more intriguing. Thus, we did expect that spending a year in Europe (and using part of that time for traveling around) would somehow influence these students' general views about Europe and the Europeans, or that it would at least affect their beliefs about the characteristics of their own nation. If such changes did occur, they were not detected with the measures employed in this study. Except for a somewhat greater reluctance to make stereotype judgments, there was little change in the dimensions of these students' "cognitive maps" of Europe, in their autostereotypes, or in their attitudes and stereotypes of other European nations.

What are the reasons for the deterioration in attitudes towards and beliefs about the host nation? Our design allows us to rule out external influences as well as regression effects and maturational changes (Campbell & Stanley, 1966). For example, if there had been some open conflict between the American and the French government that created hostility between the two nations, it should have affected the attitudes towards the French of the American students who stayed in Germany as well as of those who stayed in France. There is no evidence for such a change. Compared to the groups interviewed immediately after arrival, no significant changes could be observed in the attitudes and stereotypes towards the French of the Gl group, nor in the attitudes and stereotypes towards the Germans of the Fl group. Since regression should have affected all ratings that deviated from the mean, the fact that change was restricted to attitudes towards the host countries renders regression an unlikely explanation of our findings. Similarly, if change had been due to maturational factors, it should not have been limited to attitudes and stereotypes towards the host nation.

One final threat to validity which we need to consider is selection. As noted, only half of the population of exchange students from California State University agreed to fill out the extensive questionnaire, and we do not have information about potential differences in attitudes between accepters and refusers. However, although there is the possibility that selection operates on attitudes toward the host country, there is no obvious direction that such a bias could take. Furthermore, we can ascertain that the four groups do not show any significant differences with regard to a large set of attitude measures.

This study was less successful in pinpointing those aspects of the exchange situation which were responsible for the differences in stereotypes and/or attitudes. It was apparent that the exchange situation and particularly, the living arrangements, did offer students less opportunity to meet members of their host nation than they would have liked. Thus, more than 60% of the sample wished for better contacts. Students in both countries reported great difficulty in establishing contacts with members of the host population (student or nonstudent), but the problem seems to have been more severe in France than in Germany. Furthermore, the French were also perceived as more hostile towards Americans than the Germans. Although this could merely be a reflection of these students' greater dislike for the French, it is intriguing that the perceived attitudes of the host students correlate highly with attitudes towards the hosts in France but not Germany.

The Impact of Student Exchange Reconsidered

It is a well-documented phenomenon that people remember their own predictions incorrectly and exaggerate with hindsight what they knew beforehand (Fischhoff, 1975). Similarly, once one knows that student exchange is likely to lead to a deterioration in stereotypes and attitudes, it is difficult to remember why one should ever have expected a different outcome. It was emphasized in our description of the studies on the effect of social contact on attitudes (e.g., Cook, 1984) that the people involved in these situations were typically selected for prejudiced beliefs and attitudes. While this made it difficult to get research participants to interact in a pleasant manner, this situation has the one great advantage that there is room for improvement in their attitudes.

Students who choose to study abroad are also a highly selected group, but one selected for their positive attitudes. Although their decision seems to be mainly motivated by a wish to improve their language skill or to learn about the culture of the host country, people who dislike the French or the Germans are unlikely to decide to study in that particular country. Thus, the average attitude towards the host nation of the members of our sample is clearly on the positive side of neutral. This does not mean that there is no room for improvement, but it is certainly the case that there is even more room for deterioration.

These attitudes are based on a set of beliefs about the characteristics of the host nation as well as the host country, which is partly reflected by our measures of stereotype. Once in the foreign country, the exchange students are likely to compare their expectations with the reality they experience. If their experience is more positive than they had expected, their attitudes improve, while a negative discrepancy leads to a deterioration in attitude. This accounts for the differential impact of the exchange situation on attitudes towards various aspects of that situation.

The predominance of negative change in studies of the impact of sojourns on attitudes suggests that the sojourner is more likely to experience a negative than a positive discrepancy, and this is quite plausible for two reasons. One is relatively obvious but should still be mentioned: people with very high expectations are more likely to be disappointed than people with low expectations. Thus, if improvement in attitudes was the main goal of student exchange, one should send the xenophobics and isolationists abroad rather than students who already like a given country enough to want to go there on exchange.

The second and perhaps less obvious reason concerns the fact that studying at a foreign university can be considered a stressful life event, that is, an event in which "demands tax or exceed the individuals' adaptive resources" (Lazarus & Launier, 1978, p.296). Living in a foreign country involves much more than speaking a strange language or eating unfamiliar food or observing unfamiliar customs. As Guthrie (1975) argues, "moving into a new culture can be a profound and hard-to-describe experience. One is deprived of familiar cues and controls. The subtle, unspoken conventions that one has learned from child-hood are changed; familiar gestures take on new meanings" (p. 98). This expe-rience can result in "culture shock" (Oberg, 1960) and lead to numerous somat-ic complaints such as stomach upsets, headaches, and sweating, which are well known somatic symptoms of stress (Brislin, 1981). While Guthrie (1975) inter-prets these symptoms from a behavioral perspective as resulting from the re-moval of positive reinforcements (e. g., customary food, usual friends, social ap-proval) and the presentation of aversive stimuli (e. g., language difficulties, unfamiliar and anxious social encounters), we would argue in terms of a more cognitive approach (e. g., learned helplessness; Abramson, Seligman & Teas-dale, 1978). In this view, for the sojourner, the world has become unpredictable and uncontrollable. Perceived loss of control leads to stress and depression. Since sojourners are likely to blame their hosts and host country for their de-pression and problems they encounter, the exchange situation may be less fa-vorable to the development of positive attitudes than commonly envisaged.

Obviously, new cues and norms will be learned in time, and this learning has to occur through observation, participation, or explicit communication (Schild, 1962). Unfortunately, however, the social isolation of many sojourners makes learning about the culture through observation as well as explicit com-munication less probable (Bochner, 1972). Thus, for many exchange students, living abroad may remain a continued stress situation requiring all their coping resources, even for the mundane tasks of daily life.

What are the implications for student exchange programs? On the basis of the theoretical perspective outlined here, a number of strategies can be suggest-ed which are likely to reduce some of the negative aspects of the exchange ex-perience. There are two ways to improve the experience of the exchange stu-dent; one involves information programs and the other direct structuring of the situation. With regard to the first, it should be possible considerably to reduce the stress of going abroad through orientation programs which teach foreign students the relevant norms and conventions of the host culture. Such pro-grams could acquaint the student with the scripts for simple everyday activities. As Ben-Ari and Amir (this volume) showed, information programs can also be successful in changing an individual's attributions about, and reactions to, the host population, by presenting them with information about the host country. However, in view of the fact that exchange students stay much longer in a given country than the tourist subjects in the study of Ben-Ari and Amir, and are also likely to be better informed at the outset, the effectiveness of this type of infor-mation program in the present context is somewhat doubtful. In line with this, Selltiz et al. (1963) found attendance at an orientation program "to have negli-gible effects on attitudes as measured towards the end of the first academic year, except for a slight increase in the frequency with which generalized state-ments were qualified" (p. 217).

With regard to the second approach, a direct structuring of the situation can be used to reduce stress by facilitating the foreign students' entry into student life, and by helping them with those tasks that make the life of any new student stressful, but which are particularly difficult for a foreigner. It is one of the major support functions of the program director (with the help of the international student office at the host university) to smooth out the majority of these more bureaucratic problems. However, providing a haven of support where American students can meet each other in the office of the program director may have the unintended negative consequence of reducing the American students' motivation for contact with the host population. Since most researchers in this area (e.g., Klineberg & Hull, 1979; Selltiz et al., 1963) agree that contacts with members of the host nation are one of the important factors in facilitating positive attitude change, it is essential that the exchange setting is structured in ways that maximize contact opportunities.

Finally, we must address the question crucial in the context of this book, whether student exchange programs are likely to increase international good will and thus contribute to the reduction of international conflict. Since most of the evidence reported in this chapter indicates that the exchange experience typically leads to a deterioration in the sojourners' stereotypes and attitudes towards the host nation, the answer to this question seems to be negative. However, there are a number of reasons to qualify this conclusion.

First, the deterioration in the sojourners' attitude towards the host nation is typically only a depolarization rather than a change towards the negative. This depolarization may merely reflect an increase in the complexity of subjects' cognitive representations of the hosts nation. Due to the greater frequency of contact over a wider range of situations and a greater variety of different types of people, individuals may have developed more complex cognitive representations of this group (i.e., they use a greater number of nonredundant features to describe the outgroup). As Linville (1982) has argued, the greater the number of nonredundant features a person uses in thinking about a group, the less likely it is that this group will be perceived as consistently good or consistently bad in all respects. While this tendency to perceive a national group as good in some respects and bad in others will have a moderating effect on individuals' attitudes towards this nation, it will also make the attitude more resistant towards change. At the end of the exchange experience, these students have more information about the host nation along more dimensions. Thus, any piece of stereotype-incongruent information to which they might be exposed in future will be confronted by a vast store of congruent information in memory. As a consequence, stereotype-incongruent propaganda aimed at creating a negative view of this nation is less likely to have an impact on their stereotype than if there were fewer pieces of knowledge available (Crocker, Fiske, & Taylor, 1984).

Second, there is some doubt whether one should extrapolate from observations of the immediate impact of student exchange to the long-term effects. Although Riegel (1953) supported the plausible hypothesis that after their return the attitudes of exchange students gravitate towards those generally held by their reference groups, there are also a number of reasons to suspect that attitudes might improve over time. As mentioned earlier, students might realize after their return that the image of the home country which they used as standard in their evaluations of the host country was rather idealized. Furthermore, experiences that were evaluated negatively at the time (e.g., as strange or anxiety-arousing) may now be seen in a much more positive light (e.g., as funny or adventurous). Finally, many exchangees may come to realize in retrospect that having lived abroad is something which differentiates them positively from their more sedentary colleagues or friends (e.g., they may feel more cosmopolitan). It seems plausible that, as part of this reconstruction of their past, they will also reassess their attitude towards the former host nation. Thus, despite the evidence that the immediate impact of exchange studies on attitudes and stereotypes towards the host nation tends to be negative, it is possible that the long-term effects may be much more positive.

Finally, the assessment of the contribution of "exchange-of-person programs" to the prevention or reduction of conflict should also consider the impact of the exchange on members of the host nation. Although we could find no published data on this issue, it seems plausible that the development of personal relationships between exchange students and members of the host nation should have an impact on the relevant stereotypes and attitudes of the hosts. While the extent and direction of this change will depend on some of the same factors as determine the impact of the sojourn on attitudes of the exchange students, the fact that exchange students typically establish close contacts with a sizeable number of members of the host nation suggests that their impact on the hosts may be at least as important as the attitudinal impact of the hosts on the sojourners.

Acknowledgments. The authors would like to thank Drs. Pence, Young, and McNeal from the California State University, the Akademische Auslandsamt of Tübingen University, and the Tübinger Sprachinstitut für their support at various stages of data collection. We are also greatly indebted to Drs. Michael Diehl, Miles Hewstone, Arie Kruglanski, and Margaret Stroebe for their valuable comments on several drafts of this chapter.

References

Abramson, L. Y., Seligman, M. E. P., & Teasdale, J. D. (1978). Learned helplessness in humans: Critique and reformulation. *Journal of Abnormal Psychology, 87,* 49–74.

Allport, G. (1954). *The nature of prejudice.* Reading, MA: Addison-Wesley.

Amir, Y. (1969). Contact hypothesis in ethnic relations. *Psychological Bulletin, 71,* 319–342.

Bochner, S. (1972). Problems in culture learning. In: S. Bochner & P. Wicks (Eds.), *Overseas students in Australia.* Randwick, NSW.: New South Wales University Press.

Breitenbach, D. (1970). The evaluation of study abroad. In: I. Eide (Ed.), *Students as links between cultures.* Paris: UNESCO and the International Peace Research Institute (Oslo).

Brigham, J. C. (1971). Ethnic stereotypes. *Psychological Bulletin, 76,* 1, 15–38.

Brislin, R. W. (1981). *Cross-cultural encounters: Face-to-face interaction.* New York: Pergamon.

Campbell, D. T., & Stanley, J. C. (1966). *Experimental and quasi-experimental designs for research.* Chicago: Rand McNally.

Cantril, H. (Ed.). (1950). *Tensions that cause wars.* Urbana: University of Illinois Press.

Chang, H.-B. (1973). Attitudes of Chinese students in the United States. *Sociology and Social Research, 58,* 66–77.

Church, A.T. (1982). Sojourner adjustment. *Psychological Bulletin, 91,* 540–572.

Coelho, G.V. (1958). *Changing images of America: A study of Indian students' perceptions.* Glencoe, IL: Free Press.

Cook, S.W. (1969). Motives in a conceptual analysis of attitude-related behavior. *Nebraska symposium on motivation* (Vol 17, pp 179–235) Lincoln: University of Nebraska Press.

Cook, S.W. (1984), Cooperative interaction in multiethnic contexts. In: N.Miller, & M.B.Brewer (Eds.), *Groups in contact.* New York: Academic.

Cook, S.W., & Selltiz, C. (1955). Some factors which influence the attitudinal outcomes of personal contact. *International Social Science Bulletin, 7,* 45–51.

Crocker, J., Fiske, S.T., & Taylor, S.E. (1984). Schematic bases of belief change. In J.R.Eiser (Ed.), *Attitudinal judgment.* New York: Springer.

Deutsch, M. (1973). *The resolution of conflict.* New Haven: Yale University Press.

Deutsch, S.E., & Won, G.Y.M. (1963). Some factors in the adjustment of foreign nationals in the United States. *Journal of Social Issues, 19,* 115–122.

Fischhoff, B. (1975). Hindsight ≠ foresight: The effect of outcome knowledge on judgment under uncertainty. *Journal of Experimental Psychology: Human Perception and Performance, 1,* 288–299.

Guthrie, G.M. (1975). A behavioral analysis of culture learning. In: R.W.Brislin, S.Bochner, & W.J.Lonner (Eds.), *Cross-cultural perspectives on learning.* New York: Wiley.

Hafeez Zaidi, S.M. (1975). Adjustment problems of foreign Muslim students in Pakistan. In R.W.Brislin, S.Bochner, W.J.Lonner (Eds.), *Cross-cultural perspectives on learning.* New York: Wiley.

Hewstone, M. & Brown, R.J. (1986). Contact is not enough: An intergroup perspective on the 'contact hypothesis.' In M.Hewstone & R.J Brown (Eds.), *Contact and conflict in intergroup encounters.* Oxford. Blackwell.

Katz, D., & Braly, K.W. (1933). Racial stereotypes of one hundred college students. *Journal of Abnormal and Social Psychology, 28,* 280–290.

Klineberg, O. (1954). *Social psychology.* New York: Holt-Rinehart & Winston.

Klineberg, O. (1966). International exchanges in education, science, and culture. *Social Sciences Information, 4,* 91–143.

Klineberg, O., & Hull, W.F. (1979). *At a foreign university: An international study of adaptation and coping.* New York: Praeger.

Lazarus, R.S., & Launier, R. (1978). Stress-related transactions between person and environment. In L.A.Pervin & M.Lewis (Eds.), *Perspectives in interactional psychology.* New York: Plenum.

Linville, P.W. (1982). The complexity-extremity effect and age-based stereotyping. *Journal of Personality and Social Psychology, 42,* 193–211.

Loomis, C.P., & Schuler, E.A. (1948). Acculturation of foreign students in the United States. *Applied Anthropology, 7,* 17–34.

Lysgaard, S. (1955). Adjustment in a foreign society: Norwegian Fulbright grantees visiting the United States. *International Social Science Bulletin, 7,* 45–51.

Morris, R.T. (1960). *The two-way mirror: National status in foreign students' adjustment.* Minneapolis: University of Minnesota Press.

Oberg, K. (1960). Cultural shock. Adjustment to new cultural environments. *Practical Anthropology, 7,* 177–182.

Riegel, O.W. (1953). Residual effects of exchange-of-persons. *Public Opinion Quarterly, 17,* 319–327.

Schild, E.O. (1962). The foreign student as a stranger learning the norms of the host culture. *Journal of Social Issues, 18,* 41–54.

Selltiz, C., Christ, J.R., Havel, J., & Cook, S.W. (1963). *Attitudes and social relations of foreign students in the United States.* Minneapolis: University of Minnesota Press.

Selltiz, C., & Cook, S.W. (1962). Factors influencing attitudes of foreign students towards the host country. *Journal of Social Issues, 18,* 7–23.

Sewell, W.H., & Davidsen, O.M. (1961). *Scandinavian students on an American campus.* Minneapolis: University of Minnesota Press.

Sherif, M. (1967). *Group conflict and cooperation.* London: Routledge & Kegan Paul.

Sherif, M., Harvey, O.J., White, B.J., Hood, W.R., & Sherif, C.W. (1961). *Intergroup conflict and cooperation: The Robbers' Cave experiment*. Norman, OK: University of Oklahoma Book Exchange.

de Sola Pool, I. (1965). Effects of cross-national contact on national and international images. In H.C. Kelman (Ed.), *International behavior*. New York: Holt, Rinehart & Winston.

Spaulding, S., & Flack, M.J. (with Tate, S., Mahon, P., & Marshall, C.) (1976). *The world's students in the United States. A review and evaluation of research on foreign students*. New York: Praeger.

Stapf, K.-H., Stroebe, W. & Jonas, K. (1986). *Amerikaner über Deutschland und die Deutschen. Urteile und Vorurteile*. Opladen: Westdeutscher Verlag.

Wish, M., Deutsch, M. & Biener, L, (1970). Differences in conceptual structures of nations. An exploratory study. *Journal of Personality and Social Psychology, 16,* 361–373.

Young, F.W., & Lewycky, R. (1981). *ALSCAL-4 User's Guide. A guide for users of ALSCAL-4: A nonmetric multidimensional scaling and unfolding program with several individual differences options*. Technical report, University of North Carolina, Chapel Hill.

Author Index

Subject Index

Springer Series in Social Psychology

Springer Series in Social Psychology